Emptying Beds

EMPTYING BEDS

The Work of an Emergency Psychiatric Unit

Lorna A. Rhodes

UNIVERSITY OF CALIFORNIA PRESS
Berkeley   Los Angeles   Oxford

University of California Press
Berkeley and Los Angeles, California

University of California Press
Oxford, England

Library of Congress Cataloging-in-Publication Data

Rhodes, Lorna Amarasingham.
    Emptying beds: the work of an emergency psychiatric unit / Lorna
Amarasingham Rhodes
        p.   cm.
    Includes bibliographical references.
    Includes index.
    ISBN 0–520–07054–2 (cloth: alk. paper)
    1. Psychiatric hospitals—Emergency service—Administration.
I. Title.
    [DNLM: 1. Emergency Services, Hospital—organization &
administration.   2. Emergency Services, Psychiatric—organization &
administration.   WM 401 R476e]
RC480.6.R46   1990
362.2'1—dc20
DNLM/DLC
for Library of Congress   90–11161
                                                                    CIP

Printed in the United States of America

1 2 3 4 5 6 7 8 9

To the memory of my parents
LILLYAN JACOBS RHODES
DANIEL RHODES

Contents

Figures

Acknowledgments

Many people helped to bring this book into being. My greatest debt is to the staff of the "APU" for their willingness to include me in their reality and to take a chance on my interpretation of it. I am especially grateful to "Anthony Giuliani," who had the imagination to take me into his institution and the courage to support my work long after it had escaped our initial definition. "Sam Wishinski" is the "without whom . . . nothing" of this book; he was determined that I understand his world and spent many patient hours seeing to it that I did. "Ben Caldwell," "aberrant villager" *par excellence,* always found time to guide me through another of the unit's puzzles; the generous spirit of "Lillian Morgan" was indispensable to my incorporation into the unit's daily life. To all the staff—residents, medical students, nurses, mental health workers, and counselors—I am deeply grateful for their help and tolerance.

The Department of Psychiatry at "University" supported me both financially and psychologically during the research for this book. To the colleagues there who went out of their way to help me, and especially to those with whom I taught, I express my deep appreciation.

I want to thank the many friends and colleagues who read successive incarnations of this manuscript, especially David Spain, Stevan Harrell, Charles Leslie, Donald Light, Howard Stein, Donna Leonetti, and Erika Goldstein. Responsibility for its contents remains, of course, with me.

Part of the writing of this book was supported by a Graduate School Research Fund grant from the University of Washington, which I gratefully acknowledge.

Many friends have seen me through the years of research and writing. Emily Martin provided thoughtful comments and, more important, the inspiration that made the book seem possible. Lorraine Hunt and Andra Samelson have been steadfast fellow travelers. I have learned much from Valentine Daniel, whom I thank for his intellectual generosity and unfailing friendship. And I am grateful beyond words to Marri Parkinson for her loving presence in my life.

I thank Aaron Rhodes for his affectionate support, and Lila Amarasingham for comprehension and patience beyond her years. This book is dedicated to the memory of my parents, with love, and in gratitude for their many gifts.

Introduction

This book is about the practice of emergency psychiatry in an American city. I am concerned with how the staff of an inner-city inpatient emergency ward—charged with "managing" and "placing" the acutely distressed people who emerge from this environment—experience their work.

The nine-bed Acute Psychiatry Unit*—called the APU by its staff—and the Frederick Douglass Community Mental Health Center of which it was a part had come into being in the mid-1970s as a response to the deinstitutionalization of psychiatric patients. The intent of its founders was to provide short-term psychiatric care tailored to the immediate needs of the residents of Midway City. The psychiatrists, social workers, nurses, and aides who staffed the emergency ward were, however, in a difficult position. They worked in an environment of diminished resources and uncertain community and found themselves at the intersection of the urgent and often conflicting needs of the patients, the patients' families, the hospital, and the city.

Three aspects of the unit's work particularly captured my attention. The first was the contradictory nature of the task: the staff described themselves as having an "impossible mandate" that required that they discharge patients quickly and yet treat them adequately. The second was the way the staff lived with this contradiction: they dealt with it in strategies for action and in outrageous and ironic verbal display. Finally, I was fascinated by the self-consciousness of the staff: in their talk with me and with each other they reflected on their problematic responsibilities and on the nature of the contextual and specific knowledge they had acquired.

*The names of the people and places in this book are pseudonyms. Identifying features of people and places have also been changed. In addition, I have purposely omitted reference to the dates of the events described.

efficient but not effective

I was introduced to the unit through the clinical director of the hospital, Anthony Giuliani, who hired me to work part time in his institution. He thought that there were certain "puzzles" about the hospital that an anthropologist might be able to make sense of and that these puzzles were particularly evident in the functioning of the emergency unit. One area that concerned him was "aftercare"; he wondered whether there was some way to persuade more patients to return for outpatient appointments after they were discharged. Another puzzle was the efficiency of the emergency unit in discharging patients quickly: how, he wondered, did staff accomplish this while maintaining a generally cheerful attitude?

When I met with Sam Wishinski, the director of the emergency psychiatric unit, and Ben Caldwell, who directed the hospital's emergency services department, they seemed pleased to talk with an anthropologist. Both had spent time in other countries and had no difficulty imagining that anthropology might be a suitable perspective from which to explore the work they were doing. The first thing they told me was that their service was "opposite in all ways" to "regular" psychiatry which, in their view, "denied a whole segment of the population." Their unit operated, they said, in the "unconscious" of psychiatry. They compared themselves to the "aberrant villager" who is the first to approach the anthropologist and who, out of his alienation, is able to reveal the underside of the normal life of the village.

This was the beginning of a two-year association in which I explored with Sam, Ben, and the rest of the APU staff the relationship between the puzzles Giuliani had given me and their position in what they perceived to be psychiatry's unconscious. Eventually I realized that the puzzles could be compared to the symptoms of the "presenting patient" in a family; they were not entities amenable to objective analysis, but rather complex representations of contradictions in the situation of the hospital and its patients. These contradictions were not discrete problems that might perhaps be solved if the right social scientist could be found, but were inseparable from the active practice of those on the front line of the emergency service. The staff incorporated me into this practice, not to help them take care of their patients but to listen as they conveyed their understanding of what they were doing. Their understanding was not expressed in terms of any single or integrated meaning to be found in the work, but rather as an ongoing confrontation with ambiguity and contradiction.

Most of the material presented in this account comes from meetings of the emergency unit staff, from interviews with the staff, and from attendance on the unit, where I listened in on interviews with patients and conversations among staff members. I also met regularly with Anthony Giuliani, and I visited other parts of the system in which the unit was embedded.[1] The drawings that illustrate the text were gathered by asking the staff to "draw a picture of the unit."[2] During my study of the APU I was also involved in teaching medical students at the university with which the hospital was affiliated, an experience that contributed to my interest in the unit's training of medical students and residents.

Although I am not a clinician and was, in that sense, an outsider in relation to the activity of the unit, I participated in its practice in a way similar to that described by Jeanne Favret-Saada in her study of witchcraft in the Bocage (1980). She describes her experience of incorporation into the world of the French peasants who were her informants and notes that it was impossible to learn about witchcraft from an "outside" position, a position from which her informants' lives would appear to be a "continuous surface without holes." Instead, she had to be vulnerable herself to the "holes" in their experience that constituted the matrix in which witchcraft could make sense.

My experience of working on the APU was similar in that I understood the position of the staff through the ways in which I fell into the "holes," the vulnerable spots, in their experience. One of these was my position as an employee. I too was dependent on the hospital and administration and shared with the staff of the APU the experience of being embedded in cross-cutting and contradictory expectations. I found that I shared their perception that there was "no non-guilty position" on which to stand. For example, certain practices on the APU were questionable and perhaps illegal when seen from an outside perspective. Was my responsibility to the administration (as an employee owing allegiance to the institution and its reputation), to the staff (as an anthropologist bound to protect their confidentiality), or to the patients (as an outside observer who might be able to affect their situation)? I chose the second path (though not without considerable confusion and discomfort), waiting, listening, and trying to understand the context that made such practices, if not defensible, at least comprehensible.

My tendency to listen, to understand through silence or through shared storytelling, constitutes another "hole," a way in which my style matched that of the staff and drew me into their world. Toward the end of my study, one staff member commented:

> *You are the listener. People use you as a bridge, to feel connected to each other . . . we [each] have something to say [to you] which is part of the puzzle.*

I listened to the staff as they argued, planned, disclaimed, joked, and raged, taking as my center those who most intensely articulated their involvement with the unit. Their talk did not form a coherent "picture" of their work, and in fact they constantly warned me away from picture metaphors and overly neat conclusions. What held them together as workers was the necessity for action in the face of contradiction, and their talk reflected the discontinuity and intensity attendant on this task.

Thus, though I left the unit assuming that my task was to "connect" where the staff had not, to solve the "puzzle" by "making sense" of the unit's contradictions, I eventually realized that the contradictions *were* the sense of the unit. Many current and competing approaches to problems in mental health care "spoke" and were embedded in the voices and events I had recorded. The staff of the APU were *bricoleurs* of psychiatric and social theory, using what was available according to whether it would fit a particular context, drawing upon what Ingleby calls the "bewildering array of theoretical approaches" (1983:142) to fit their pragmatic orientation. At any moment, and sometimes all in the same moment, a staff member might be a biological empiricist, a Freudian, or a Laingian antipsychiatrist. The unit was, as a friend of mine put it, a place of "patches without a quilt" where immediate problems could be seen in any number of ways, none of which added up to a frame that would bring the whole into coherence. I have not used any particular theory from within psychiatry or social psychiatry to discuss the situation I describe. Rather, I hope that the unit will function for the reader, as it has for me, to reveal multiple and contradictory perspectives. I have tried to convey the unit's polyphonic and concrete interplay of voices, along with my own sensation of immersion in it as a listener and co-speaker.

One way of looking at psychiatry emphasizes the patients it treats; the questions center on what is wrong with them (and this can be framed in many ways, from biological to psychodynamic to familial theories of causation), what should be done for them, and what effect they have on those treating them. From this perspective, though the problems may be numerous and intractable, the issue of agency is fairly straightforward; those who treat psychiatric patients/problems are trying to help them to attain lives of greater functioning and ease. Much of the literature generated by psychiatry itself assumes this perspective and treats many of the problems of psychiatric settings (for example, the emotional negativity therapists may feel toward patients, or the entanglement of psychiatry with the legal system) as interfering with their basic mission. The question is how to overcome these obstacles in the interest of the patient.

Another perspective, often considered antagonistic to the first, considers psychiatrists and other practitioners as "agents of social control"

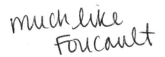
much like Foucault

whose primary role is to contain deviance and preserve the social order. David Ingleby sums up this perspective thus:

> *[The] "critical view" argues that "mental illness" is to a large extent socially caused, or even socially constructed; that the goal of treatment has to do with the maintenance of social order, . . . and that the domination of the medical profession is neither warranted nor desirable. (1983:143)*

Views on the ways in which illness is socially constructed and on the nature of medical domination vary widely within this perspective, but there is general agreement that psychiatric professionals are the agents of forces that are not, at bottom, in the interests of the patient. The "treatment agent" is to some extent an actor (consciously or unconsciously) in the interests of a larger system, whether it be professional practice (Light 1980; Scull 1979) political economy (Scull 1979; Warner 1985) or "society," rather vaguely conceived as an agglomeration of controlling individuals (Szaz 1961; Scheff 1966). Therapy may be represented as a medical or humanitarian necessity, but its real function is to control, contain, or remove from society those who threaten or overburden it. *discipline and punish*

Both the therapeutic and the social control perspective are useful; the first draws attention to the complexity of subjective experience, whereas the second makes us aware of the larger social context in which subjectivity takes shape. But both take on a different coloring when approached from within a psychiatric institution. Many writers on institutional settings have found that the world of patients and staff defies explanation in terms of either mental illness or society. Young psychiatrists are inaugurated into work that is full of ambiguity and mystification (Light 1980; Coser 1979) and patients are caught between resistance and collusion (Caudill 1957; Estroff 1981; Goffman 1961; Reynolds 1977). The institution reveals itself to be constituted of "binds"—ambiguous relationships between form and content, constraint and opportunity—to which practitioners respond in pragmatic and strategic ways. From the perspective of those who work in institutions, the tension between context and agency is ongoing and irresolvable; it emerges continually in action and is resolved in actions that, in turn, bring further tension. Resistance and acquiescence are perpetually in balance (cf. Comaroff 1985; Ortner 1984).

The work of Michel Foucault has been important in my thinking about these aspects of institutional life. Foucault writes about institutions not merely as places that reflect or contain larger societal problems, but as "figures" (Lentricchia 1988:84) for the fundamental ways in which society and institution mirror and shape one another. In his studies of

Rhodes doesn't think emptying beds is effective

the asylum, the hospital, and the prison, Foucault shows that in the late eighteenth and early nineteenth century the inner space of these institutions developed a configuration that provided for the development of the peculiarly modern relationship between subject and object; through the manipulation and management of the body, the inmate became an object of knowledge and a subject of discipline (1973; 1979).

My intention in this book is not to provide an analysis or critique of the work of Foucault. Rather, I want to use Foucault's notions of disciplinary space, power/knowledge, and subjectivity to illuminate the work of the APU. The similarities I found between the talk of the staff and the writings of Foucault are surely not accidental; the APU staff speak from the center of the kind of disciplinary space Foucault describes and describe themselves enmeshed in precisely the ambiguous relationship between subject and object that such a space produces. Thus I see the APU as a "field" in a larger sense than that usually implied in the notion of anthropological "field" work (though Foucault suggests historical kinship between the terms). The APU is a field of power in Foucault's sense, where certain fundamental "mechanisms" of our society are visible. It is precisely these mechanisms that remain opaque if the psychiatric hospital is considered a "small society" (Caudill 1957) operating according to principles of social organization incorporated from sociology or psychology.

APU = field of power in F's sense

In allowing Foucault and the APU staff to serve as commentaries for one another, my emphasis is not only on the patients constructed as objects by the staff but also on the ways in which the staff themselves were made subjects of discipline. The notion that the staff were enmeshed in a space in which they were both watchers and watched, disciplining and disciplined, helps us to see the complex and paradoxical nature of their situation.

Part of the paradox lies in the nature of the staff's power. Power, as Foucault shows, does not rest in the hands of individuals or groups; rather it is fluid and diffuse, operating in a net-like grid of relationships. This analogy to a net or web corresponds to my observation of the way the unit worked. The staff did not employ a single kind of power (as, for example, the power to label patients as mentally ill, or, conversely, the power to make them well), nor did they use their powers in a clear, unidirectional way. Moreover, the patients were not passive in the face of power. Rather, administrators, staff, and patients were engaged in a situation of shifting, reciprocal, and multidirectional power relations. I do not mean by this that the unit's staff did not exercise more power than the patients; they did. But in order to understand the nature of clinical practice on the unit, we cannot depend for explanation on a "power-over" arrow that points only from the staff to the patients or, for that matter, from the the state or the economy to the staff. Rather, staff, patients, administrators, and other institutions have to be seen as bound together in the same disciplinary space, one in which all, to varying degrees, are subjects of power.

The staff of the APU did not accede passively to their enmeshment in a system of power. "Where there is power there is resistance" (Foucault 1978:95) and they found ways to resist, through strategy, humor, and subversion of discipline. The resistance of the staff was covert, ephemeral, and oblique;[3] it served to throw into relief, at every turn, ways in which the work constantly threatened to become absurd. Many of the "techniques for making useful individuals" that pervaded the hospital—from the patient interview to the writing of charts—had the potential to be subverted or mocked. This subversion was not peripheral to the "real" work of clinical practice, something that would end were the institution to be retooled to more perfectly meet the needs of its constituents. It was part and parcel of the work itself, and to the extent that the work had meaning to the staff it was because they made something tangible out of their experience of disjunction, contradiction, and absurdity. Novels and popular accounts of clinical work sometimes make this point indirectly, as when, in *The House of God* (Shem 1978) the intern/antihero is asked by those outside the hospital how he can laugh about what he is doing. The APU staff pointed out that the same dynamic is at work in television shows that exploit the paradoxical and absurd character of institutional work.

Like the protagonists of these books and comedy shows, the APU staff felt that their workplace was special and unique, set apart from an outside world that could not understand or respond to it. In their view the practice required a collusion and deviousness that concealed the particular and pragmatic character of their understanding from those who would incorporate it into normal institutional mechanisms. Elizabeth Traube mentions that during her fieldwork in a remote part of the island of Timor she believed, with her informants, that they were presenting her with a special knowledge that alone would enable her to make sense of their history (1986:243). Later she realized that their very insistence on the specialness of their knowledge was part of that history. Similarly, I felt while I was on the APU that I was being asked to attend to a peculiar and unusual way of thinking about the world of clinical work. Now, however, I believe that this impression was a result of the staff's attempt to convey an understanding rooted in local and specific circumstances—what Foucault calls "subjugated knowledge"—and to contrast this with the standardized knowledge produced by objectification within disciplinary space. The local knowledge of the staff was highly contextual, strategic, and personal. It contrasted with (and made

actors' methods of efficiency are not necessarily effective

strategic use of) the knowledge of diagnosis, treatment, administration, law, and management that constituted the more visible aspects of the institution. The difference between these kinds of knowledge—often brought out as a contrast between what could be said and what had to be written—lies behind many episodes of conflict or resistance described in this book.

Foucault insists that his task is not to provide intellectual comfort in the face of discomfiting social realities. Rather than offering a specific critique based on the idea that it is possible to reject "all possible solutions except for the one valid one," he suggests that we approach social problems in a spirit of "problematization" that leaves the door open for original, unconventional, or radical understanding. He says,

> [my attitude is] more on the order of "problematization"—which is to say, the development of a domain of acts, practices, and thoughts that seem to me to pose problems for politics. For example, I don't think that in regard to madness and mental illness there is any "politics" that can contain the just and definitive solution. But I think that in madness, in derangement, in behavior problems, there are reasons for questioning politics. (1984:385)

Perhaps more important for this account than any particular insight of Foucault into the nature of institutions is this insistence on the need for problematization. It seems to me that when the staff of the APU recognized the potentially subversive nature of my writing—the fact that my notebook recorded their speech—and yet continued to encourage it, they wanted me to attend to their problematization of their situation. They insisted that I not foreclose on what they were doing, that I not assume that even the theories they were fond of could provide solutions to their dilemmas. I have tried to retain this spirit of problematization, keeping to the sense of ambiguity and lack of closure that was vividly expressed to me.

I want to point out three areas in particular that are deliberately problematized in this account. First, and most important, are the patients. The voices of the unit's patients appear here only as they were heard by, and in relation to, the unit's staff. I do not pretend to represent the patients "as they were"—that would require a different book—but rather as they appeared to the staff. At times the patients were objects to be sorted, held, and then disposed of. At other times particular patients became symbolic of specific dilemmas in the unit's operation. Some patients came to be representations of, and repositories for, emotions of anger, disgust, compassion, or love. And occasionally the staff arrived at what seemed an almost existential acceptance of the patients as representative, in their very poverty and craziness, of the human condition. Estroff says of the outpatients she worked with that "it is too easy to avoid or to oversimplify [their] human, often tragic dimension . . . And it is persuasively simplistic to stress the tragedy and to overlook the essentially bittersweet, paradoxical nature of these lives" (1985:198). In reproducing the multiple, inconsistent, and self-conscious ways in which APU staff responded to patients, and in allowing the patients to appear in this book in the same partial and incomplete way that they appeared on the unit, I too hope that the bittersweet of their lives shows through.

Second, I problematize psychiatry. Psychiatry is not the subject of this book, but rather one of its protagonists. Psychiatry appears in the form of goals, diagnoses, medications, and explanations, but these do not add up to a picture that represents or distorts some ideal type of psychiatric practice. Perhaps a useful analogy is the difference, in complex societies like India, between the great and the little traditions. In the context of work on the APU, psychiatry and psychoanalysis are great traditions that provide the rules, vocabulary, and mythology from which the little tradition draws (cf. Marriott 1955). Of course, in fact, the great tradition itself is changeable and historically situated. But the point here is that the little tradition is not a direct reflection of a great tradition; rather, it takes from the great tradition what is useful, and often uses it in local, context-specific ways. This could be seen on the APU in the way diagnoses, taken from the "sacred text" of the *Diagnostic and Statistical Manual of Mental Disorders, Third Edition* (APA 1980), were put to strategic uses entirely bound up with the immediate needs of the unit. It could also be seen in the ways the vocabulary of psychoanalysis was called into service for the description of emotion, providing a way to place emotion where it could best be dealt with at any given moment. In portraying the psychiatric side of the APU's practice I have tried to remain as much as possible within the little tradition perspective of the unit itself; psychiatry constituted some of the stuff with which the quilt patches of the unit's work were constructed, but not a larger explanatory focus that would provide a whole quilt to put them in. In *Reflection in Action* Schön suggests that many settings for professional work are like swamps in which practitioners must find their own path, using an intuitive, reflective approach to practice that may be guided by, but cannot directly match, the profession's texts and traditions (1983). The APU was such a swamp; in what one staff member called the unit's "moral murk," psychiatry was refracted and fragmented, and the fragments were then used to illuminate the path.

Finally, this account problematizes issues of agency and subjectivity and, in the process, Foucault's description of totalizing institutions. In disciplinary space as it is described in *Discipline and Punish* it seems that subjectivity is entirely shaped, imprinted, and normalized (1979; cf.

Lentricchia 1988). Historical and subjective agency is a delusion; the mechanisms that give institutions their distinctive character as loci of power relations shape the inner life of individuals, who find themselves in "an iron cage worse than any Weber ever dreamed of" (Berman 1982:35). But it seems to me that in giving us a figure that images power as both pervasive and fluid and that insists on the intrinsic character of resistance, Foucault also suggests that disciplinary space has chinks and crannies in which we can, if we will, recover the possibility of agency. In a later interview he says that his intent is to show "the arbitrariness of institutions and . . . which space of freedom we can still enjoy and how many changes can still be made" (Martin et al. 1988:11).

Mary Pratt points out that in contrast to the objective seeing of science, "subjective experience . . . is spoken from a moving position already within or down in the middle of things, looking and being looked at, talking and being talked at" (1986:32). The APU staff and patients were "within and down in the middle" of their work, as was I when I studied them, and their subjectivity is expressed throughout this book. This is particularly evident in the emotional tone of much of what is recorded here; the anger, humor, and frustration voiced by the staff should not be reduced to easy formulas (e.g., stress or denial) but allowed to stand as expressions of fundamental dilemmas in their position (cf. Hahn 1985:56). Similarly, the centrality of particular individuals in this account—funny, difficult, and inconsistent as they are—suggests the way the staff tried to make a mark on their environment. What is problematic is whether this agency mattered. Was it, as Foucault said of the writing of early psychiatric reformers, "so much incidental music" (1973), swallowed up by the disciplinary agenda of the institution? Or was the expressive life of the staff, flowering in whatever chinks it found, somehow providing the ground for a new kind of criticism? Throughout this study, I have tried to convey the way the issue remained in balance.

ONE

Starkness Was Everywhere

I

The whole world is a mental hospital and I've been locked up all my life.

—A Patient

"TOUCH me YOU will DIE, TOUCH me YOU will DIE, TOUCH me YOU will DIE, TOUCH me YOU will DIE . . ." A man has entered the Frederick Douglass Center and stands in the doorway between the screening area and the Acute Psychiatry Unit. The admitting nurse rolls her eyes and wearily punches the button for Security. A few staff members move calmly toward the area, seemingly unimpressed with the enormous size and threatening manner of the new arrival.

Two security officers arrive.

"What do you want us to do?" one asks a nearby mental health worker.

"What should we do?" the mental health worker asks a nearby nurse.

The nurse in turn asks, "Where's Sally?"

"Trying to pull towels out of the toilet in Nine."

"For Christ's sake, she should be here."

Just then a door opens into the screening room and a thin, wispy sixty-year-old woman, looking very like a nun, enters carrying a sopping white towel with the Douglass Center logo.

"TOUCH me YOU will DIE, TOUCH me YOU will DIE, TOUCH me YOU will DIE . . ." continues the enormous man.

"Look at this, just look at this," shouts the nun. "I feel like wringing this around Jimmie's neck. That's the last time I let him have a room with a bathroom. I told him, 'Jimmie, next time I see you, you better know how to piss in a bag, because I'll be goddamned if I let you in a bathroom again.'"

"Sally, what do you want us to do with this guy?"

"What guy? We're drowning back there, pretty soon we'll need gondolas to get to the day room, and you ask me what to do with somebody. Anyway, there aren't any beds on the unit. The only bed is on Five West."

Everyone groans. From the guards to the mental health aides, everyone knows that Five West isn't a solution. The huge man continues implacably.

"Sam will have to transfer someone," says Sally.

One of the staff pushes open another door. Inside, a resident, two medical students, and a social worker are standing around a bespectacled psychiatrist whose thinning hair and bushy beard make him vaguely reminiscent of Groucho Marx.

"Did you get Housekeeping?" Sally shouts through the door.

"They're short-staffed today but they're sending down some dinghies and life preservers," Sam replies.

"Good, then you take this man here and put him back there," says Sally, gesturing to the man in the doorway.

"How the hell can I do that? I don't have any beds." Sam walks out of the screening area, looks at the man, walks back into the nurses' station and says to the social worker, "This is it, a gift from heaven! Now we can get rid of Cunningham."

Everyone's eyes light up. Sam calls Five West and asks for Dr. Hudson.

"Hi, Barney," he says. "We understand you have a bed open, and we have a patient here who would make an excellent training case for one of your residents. Do any of them happen to know martial arts? . . . No, don't worry, he's mostly bark. Listen, you can hear him now in the background." Sam points the phone toward the chanting man and makes conductor-like movements for a crescendo, which, to everyone's amazement, he provides.

"Look, Barney," Sam continues, "I didn't invite this fellow in here. All I know is he's here and we don't have any beds . . . Transfer? You want me to transfer one of our patients to you so we can take this one?"

Staff are now so intent on this interaction that the large man is momentarily silent. Sam motions him to continue.

"Look, Barney, the only patient I could even consider sending you is one I know you wouldn't want . . . you know, the Cunningham woman I told you about the other day . . . You will? Well, are you sure? OK, if you insist, we'll send her right up." He puts down the phone with a broad smile of satisfaction. The social worker does a little dance.

The guards start toward the chanter but Sally motions them away. She has already drawn up 10 mg of haloperidol in a syringe. She waves the syringe at Sam, who nods, and she says to the man in the doorway, "Here's something to make you feel calmer. It will sting for just a moment." Apparently untroubled by the enormous difference between the patient's size and her own, she quickly administers the shot. As though it works instantaneously, the man stops his now faltering chant and follows Sally through the wet passage to the unit.

As the guards drift back to their station and the medical students retreat to their alcove behind the nursing station, Sam looks down to find a man stretched out full length at his feet. Black, disheveled, and atrociously pockmarked, he has his hands extended in a silent gesture of supplication. This is King James, a patient so familiar that his most outrageous attempts to gain readmission call forth only a tired smile. A nurse steps up to him, lifts him up by the arms, and says, "Oh, King, how did you get back here?" She takes him into Screening, searches out his bulging chart, and begins the process of admission.

Now the floor is empty (except for a little trickle of water) and the phones are quiet. The unit settles into a lull of peaceful inactivity.

This is a description of a moment in the life of the Acute Psychiatry Unit. It is not, however, a scene that I recorded. Sam Wishinski, the unit's director, wrote this vignette as the opening scene of this book. Condensing many of the central features of work on the APU, it also expresses his recognition of himself and other staff members as actors in my account.

The three patients described or referred to in this incident each represent one aspect of the unit's work. The "chanter" is an "emergency" patient, one whose behavior has become so disruptive that he cannot be tolerated either in his own social world or in most medical and psychiatric settings; the staff react almost casually to his behavior, demonstrating that this kind of situation is routine to them. "King James" is a "repeating" patient, who returns to the unit frequently (suggested by his "bulging chart") and wants to be readmitted. "The Cunningham woman" is old and both mentally and physically ill: she is a "difficult" patient, "one you wouldn't want," for whom the staff of the APU have been unable to find a placement. Each of these patients poses a different problem for the staff, but they share one characteristic; no other place wants them. The focus of Sam's description is not the condition or treatment of these patients, but what they represent for the staff as objects of practice. The situation described here, repeated daily in different forms, arose from a fundamental contradiction in the unit's work: patients who needed admission created pressure to discharge patients already on the unit. The unit was designed for patients like the "chanter"—acutely ill and probably in need of brief hospitalization. But many patients, like King James, the Cunningham woman, and perhaps, in fact, the chanter himself, could not easily be "referred" because there were few places for them to go. Thus, the staff experienced constant pressure on their beds and the constant threat of a bottleneck within the unit that would make these beds unavailable to "emerging" patients. Their work can be described in terms of an implicit expectation: they had to produce empty beds.

This scene is written, then, to reflect what staff perceived to be primary to their work: strategy in the service of disposition. Workers on the unit took pride in the efficiency with which they could discharge patients. Sam's maneuver in trading the Cunningham woman for the chanter (who was likely, despite his apparent fierceness, to be easier to treat and to place)[1] displays the elements that contributed to this pride: the cunning required to outmaneuver another facility, and the ability to take the startling behavior of patients in stride and even enjoy it. Also characteristic of the unit is the fact that this episode takes place in front of medical students; part of the function of the unit was teaching, and part of what was taught was the "how to" of moving patients out. Sam makes a play on this teaching function when he describes the chanter to Dr. Hudson as "an excellent training case."

The reader may have noticed that in fact only one patient is discharged while two are admitted. This oversight on Sam's part indicates another contradiction in the unit's operation. Repeating patients presented a different kind of challenge to the staff; they indicated by their return that their previous admission and discharge were only a temporary solution to the kinds of problems that brought them to the unit. The casual readmission of James, despite the fact that the unit "had no beds"[2] results from a process of extending and redefining the unit's function as an emergency facility. A "repeater" calls for a response different, though no less matter-of-fact, than that accorded the acute or "emergent" patient.

Sam conveys a picture of the unit as a place of contrasts. Frequent and sudden shifts from hectic activity to calm resulted from the contrast between the "emergent" nature of patients' behavior and the disciplined and regulated structure of the unit's space and time. The juxtaposition of deprivation and whimsy was also a major feature of the unit's atmosphere. The context is one of scarcity; there are not enough beds, not enough services (Housekeeping hasn't unclogged the drains), and not enough places for patients to go. The patients themselves represent extremes of poverty, illness, and despair. Yet the tone of the story is whimsical; Sally makes the most of Jimmy's recalcitrance, Sam and the rest of the staff enjoy their victory over Dr. Hudson, and the angry patient is incorporated into a joke. This contrast was a major component in the self-consciousness of the staff.

Early in my study Sam echoed the question that had been posed to me by Giuliani: "How do we get these patients out so fast?" The first reason, he said, was that "the place is a hole," so unpleasant that patients want to leave. The staff felt that part of their task was to use this advantage. The other reason was what he called "indirection and deviousness," the use of strategy to achieve disposition. The staff had learned to make the most of their position at the intersection of contradictory demands, playing off needs and places against one another and succeeding, usually, in enjoying their own skill. This chapter explores the "hole" of the APU—its internal structure and the reflection of this structure in the working relationships of the staff. In the next chapter I will turn to the patients and the field of potential dispositions within which the unit was situated.

II

And yet, he [the urban developer] did not really wipe out the ashes, only moved them to another site. For the ashes are part of us.

—MARSHALL BERMAN (1982:312)

How are you going to get across fluidity when things look so concrete on paper?

—BEN CALDWELL

The Douglass Center was large (one hundred beds) and served an extensive downtown area of Midway City. This area encompassed white and black middle-class enclaves, several white, ethnic working-class neighborhoods, and a mostly black inner-city area that was suffering the dislocations of urban renewal. Most Douglass Center patients came from the black and white working-class neighborhoods of the area; lacking insurance or other resources, these patients relied on the hospital and its outlying satellite mental health centers both for help in emergencies and for ongoing support in chronic illness.

The center was located in the inner-city part of its catchment area, close to a large medical school/hospital complex and on the edge of a poor black neighborhood, much of which was destroyed by riots in the 1960s and had been rebuilt as projects. Many of the surrounding streets had the disorderly, threatening quality of urban landscapes that have been torn down and never fully rebuilt. Others were in the process of being transformed into highways, or were becoming the site of the University's expansion. A few streets around the hospital were "gentrifying" as young professionals moved in and renovated old houses. All of these developments impinged upon the people served by the center; living in projects or tenements, they were the most vulnerable to the changes in the urban landscape. Sometimes their very presence was seen as a threat to the integrity of that landscape; when the president was scheduled to visit the city, the APU staff complained that the police brought to the hospital an unusually high number of merely disreputable characters.

The center occupied a new eight-story building designed in a bland, modern style that made it resemble an office building. The building had a large front entrance with glass doors opening from the street onto a spacious lobby; these doors, however, had been sealed shut against the street. The "real" entrance was now through a small side door off the parking lot which was guarded by a gate and a security officer.

This shift in entrances, obvious to anyone entering the building, bespoke the change in attitude which had occurred since its construction less than ten years before. At that time it was planned as a "community" facility that was to be open to easy access for meetings, films, and perhaps even swimming by the public. But close contact with the underbelly of the city proved costly, and it had been "sealed" from the depradations of that same public. Thus the building presented an oddly ambiguous facade: one side, walled with big glass windows and double swinging doors, faced the city, but was shut against it; the other side, facing a covered parking area and without windows, admitted through a narrow entrance, only those who could prove that they belonged inside.

The Acute Psychiatry Unit was on the first floor of the Douglass Center, just to the right of the guarded entrance and adjacent to an emergency door wide enough to admit a police van. Near the guard's desk at the entrance was the screening area, where patients were processed when they first arrived at the hospital. Next to the screening area was "the unit," which consisted of a nurses' station, several offices, and a long, locked corridor that faced the patients' rooms. The unit had nine single rooms, each sparsely furnished with a bed and desk. There were two seclusion rooms, identical to the patient rooms and furnished only with mattresses. All the rooms had peepholes in the doors and could be locked only from the outside. At the end of the corridor of patient rooms was the day room where patients spent most of their time. No natural light entered the unit; the few windows faced from the patients' rooms onto a dark parking area and were covered with heavy screen. Near the police entrance was a small room with a shower and tub, called the "Kwell room" after the shampoo that was used there to remove lice from incoming patients.

Few personal touches could be seen on the unit. In the nurses' station a poster of a sunset read "The Sun Will Set Without Thy Assistance." The sole decoration in Sam's office was a poster that showed an old man in ragged clothes, obviously a "street person," wearing a pair of new running shoes; it was captioned "When The Going Gets Tough The Tough Get Going." An essay by Robert Louis Stevenson entitled "On the Enjoyment of Unpleasant Places" was pinned to the bulletin board. In the social workers' office, pictures cut from magazines were pasted to the walls, these scenes of mountain and ocean landscapes a contrast to the bare hallway outside.

Otherwise, the unit was devoid of decoration or embellishment. Everything, from the file cabinets and chartholders to the bare but adequate patient rooms, was functional and simple. The day room was windowless, with concrete-block walls. An old black and white television was mounted on one wall. A bookshelf held some five-year-old *Woman's Day* magazines; patients sat and had their meals at two long metal tables. On the wall was a "schedule of activities" that listed such events as "morning group" and "milieu therapy." A short acquaintance with the unit revealed this to be a phantom schedule; the real one entailed, simply enough, three meals, medication times, and bedtime. Meals were delivered to a door opening from the day room onto the lobby and were served to the patients from plastic trays. Patients lined up to receive their medication at the door to the nurses' station.

The doors of the unit were locked. Patients were locked inside and the staff, without exception, carried their own keys to the patient area. The locked doors made the patients' area a separate domain—isolated, potentially dangerous, and accessible only to those who belonged there. The APU differed from a locked ward in which the whole ward—nurses' station, offices, and conference rooms as well as patient areas—is surrounded by locked doors. On such wards the staff may "run into" and talk with patients in the course of carrying out their daily activities. On the APU, however, the nurses' station and other staff areas were separate from and outside the locked part of the unit. This separation had the effect of making entrance into the patients' area a deliberate act; the staff rarely interacted casually with patients. This architectural isolation of the patients in their locked domain reinforced the definition of the unit as a holding area for emergencies—situations that had to be radically contained, but only briefly.

The locked door that separated the nurses' station from the patients did not provide an absolute separation. Next to it was a large window. Through it the patients could watch the staff as they went about their work, and the staff could watch the patients as they paced, gestured, stared, or demanded cigarettes, coffee, or their freedom. This window was a focal point of the unit, the source of one of its nicknames: "the aquarium."

The APU was open twenty-four hours a day and employed a staff of thirty people. The mental health workers and the nurses worked in shifts, the social workers, counselors, and residents worked nine to five, and the psychiatrists were employed part-time. In this study I focus on the day shift and on the interaction among those directly involved in the disposition of patients. I will "name" fourteen staff members representing a variety of staff positions; when other members of the staff need to be mentioned I will refer to them by their position as "nurse," or "resident."[3]

Ben Caldwell was the psychiatrist who directed the evaluation and screening department within which the APU operated. Ben had been the first director of the unit and was the person most responsible for its style. Even though he no longer participated in the actual management of the unit, his presence was always felt in the background. A short, energetic man, Ben had a cool, sardonic way of talking which sometimes concealed the twinkle in his eyes. Ben was fascinated by emergency work and was not planning an eventual practice with a middle-class clientele; even after he had left the clinic, he remarked, characteristically, "I will always work with revolting patients."

Sam Wishinski directed the unit and was responsible, legally and practically, for its patients and its day to day operation. As he described himself to me at the beginning, he looked a little like Groucho Marx; bearded, balding, and intense, he walked with the help of a cane. Younger and less experienced in public psychiatry than Ben, Sam was a student at the Midway City Analytic Institute and had a private practice in an upper-middle-class suburb.

Lillian Morgan was the social worker. Vivid, outgoing, and articulate, she was an expert at the unit's most important function: finding places to which patients could be discharged. She had a shrewd grasp of the intricate world of outside resources and a blunt, no-nonsense approach to the problems of patients. A second social worker worked with Lillian; sometimes social work students rotated through the unit.

Walter Boyd was the counselor who specialized in alcoholism and addiction. He worked in the screening area of Emergency Services, but was a frequent presence on the unit. Walter combined a quick sense of humor with a sometimes bitter realism about the prospects of his patients.

The psychiatric resident was Duane Powers. On the unit for his six-month "rotation" as part of his training in psychiatry, he made many of

---

STAFF OF THE APU

ANTHONY GIULIANI	Clinical Director of the Hospital
BEN CALDWELL	Director of Emergency Services
SAM WISHINSKI	Director of the APU
LILLIAN MORGAN	Social Worker
WALTER BOYD	Counselor
DUANE POWERS	Resident
RONNIE LENAHAN	Nurse
SALLY MORROW	Nurse
ROBERT NAUMANN	Forensic Social Worker
PAUL GODDARD	Mental Health Worker
TRINA THORNE	Mental Health Worker
BARBARA WILSON	Nursing Director
BEA RADNOR	In-Patient Director
NANCY ALTMAN	Secretary

THE STAFF OF THE APU

the day to day decisions about medication and discharge. He was intelligent, conscientious, and quick-witted; within his first few weeks on the unit he had grasped the essentials of the place and forged his own style—a tough-minded efficiency softened by an often poignant sense of humor. Duane was one of several residents and many medical students who rotated through the unit while I was there. Their rotations constituted the "seasons" of the unit; in January and July, when both the resident and the medical students were new, there was a sometimes tense period of adjustment during which permanent staff made a deliberate effort to convey the nature of the work.

Ronnie Lenahan was the nurse who managed the day shift on the unit. She loved flamboyant clothes and spicy food; she usually took pleasure in the quirkiness of the patients. She also had a steady head in a crisis and was a master of the unit's paperwork.

The nurse described in Sam's opening scene was Sally Morrow. Nearing retirement, she appeared to be quiet and "wispy," but no one had a better feel for the workings of the hospital. Sally could guide a new resident through the intricacies of the admissions process and tell him what medication to give without his ever realizing that he wasn't managing by himself.

Barbara Wilson was the nurse chairperson in charge of the nursing service on the unit. A veteran of both community work and the state hospitals, she was involved largely with the administrative side of the unit's operation.

Robert Naumann was the social worker in charge of the forensic side of the hospital's work. He did not work on the unit, but came in regularly as a consultant on cases sent from the court system. Tall and often somber in his demeanor, he applied a shrewd and ready wit to the sometimes pathetic, sometimes alarming records of the forensic patients.

Two mental health workers are named here. Paul Goddard was a sturdy, friendly young man. Bitter about the dead-end nature of his job, he nevertheless took seriously the needs of the unit for male mental health workers (the unit had to have one male worker on each shift in case physical restraint was needed). Trina Thorne had been with the unit from its inception and was the mainstay of the day room. She was fascinated by horse racing and spent much of her day dividing her attention between the patients and certain elaborate calculations she carried out with the aid of racing bulletins.

Two other people were important on the unit although they do not appear frequently in the talk recorded in this book. Nancy Altman was the secretary who managed the immense quantity of paperwork the unit generated. Bea Radnor directed the inpatient service of the hospital. She did not figure in the day to day management of the unit but intervened in crises.

Anthony Giuliani, the clinical director of the hospital, was in charge of many other wards and clinics and preoccupied with the complex relationship between the hospital, the state, and the community. He was close to Ben Caldwell and knew that the unit's staff were struggling to find realistic ways to think about their work, but he was not involved in the details of the unit's daily operation. Thoughtful, sophisticated, and highly educated, Giuliani had a passionate, sometimes painful concern for the hospital's patients; he expressed intense outrage when questionable practices came to his attention.

Officially, the staff were organized into parallel hierarchies; each discipline answered to a separate line of command which extended outside the unit to the administration of the hospital—the nurses to the nurse chairperson and then to the nursing coordinator, the social workers to the hospital's social work director, and the psychiatrists to Giuliani. Within the unit, however, the staff were organized into temporary "teams," consisting of one person from each discipline, around individual patient cases. This organization created cross-cutting hierarchies and allegiances, resulting in a complex network of relationships on the unit.

The staff were also divided between those who worked on "screening" and those who worked on the "unit." "Screening," the area just inside the side entrance to the hospital, was where all patients came when they first arrived; it was staffed by residents and nurses who had the task of conducting an initial interview and deciding whether to admit or refer a patient. Only 15 percent of the patients who came through screening were admitted to the hospital. The boundary between screening and the unit was not fixed; at times, when the screening area was busy, the staff of the unit kept their door closed and remained close to their patients; at other times, especially during "lulls," the screening and unit staff made free use of one another's space. On weekends when the unit was relatively quiet and fewer people were working, the two areas blended into one; when Sally was working on weekends she often brought in lunch or dinner for everyone who was on duty.

My research on the unit lasted two years. When I began my study Sam had been its director for over a year; he left for another job a few months before I did. I have written this account to reflect the "middle period" of Sam's tenure, describing other staff members as they were at that time. Though this allows me to depict the attitudes of staff as they developed during this period, it does not convey the extent to which the unit was in flux. The staff constantly emphasized to me that the place was changeable and unstable. The rhythm of the rotation schedule ensured that there were always new faces, new students, and residents who had to learn the attitudes and practices of the permanent staff; there were also less predictable changes in the permanent staff, particularly the nurses. By the time I left, the unit had been influenced by staffing changes and administrative changes that substantially influenced its orientation to patients. Thus, in fact, things do "look more concrete on paper" than they really were.

III

Is it surprising that prisons resemble factories, schools, barracks, hospitals, which all resemble prisons?

—Michel Foucault (1979:228)

Command over money, command over space and command over time form independent but interlocking sources of social power.

—David Harvey (1985:1)

The architecture and scheduling of the APU firmly separated the staff from the patients, creating a space of confinement in which patients were enclosed, watched, and subjected to an almost unvarying routine.

The staff guarded and managed this space, but they, too, were observed and scheduled; their command over space and time varied depending on the nature of their position in the hierarchy of hospital work. At the same time the staff perceived both their own and the patients' space to be out of sight of the administration and anomalous within psychiatry and thus only partially subject to the rules that appeared to regulate the unit.

The staff called the nurses' station and screening area the "front" of the unit. The rooms, day room, and hallway inside the locked area were the "back." Though there were a couple of staff offices along the back hallway, this area was perceived as belonging to the patients and the mental health workers and was associated with confinement and low status. The addiction counselor, Walter Boyd, described it as a prison, saying that sometimes "patients from jail would rather be in jail, where there's more freedom." Paul, one of the aides who spent his days locked up in the back with the patients said, "It's a dungeon, of course; it's dark and you can't get out!" To Ronnie, the unit was "a submarine" that had "no light, and a control room." Anthony Giuliani, describing how the unit was different from other wards in the hospital, said "The whole unit is a seclusion room." Sam referred to the unit as a "perverse monastery."

These are images of "disciplinary space," suggestive of the features that are shared by prisons, hospitals, and factories. The unit shared with the prison a cellular, partitioned structure; it was a locked enclosure separated into individual rooms, each with a peep hole in the door and no lock on the inside. This space was designed to foster "time-tables, compulsory movements, regular activities, solitary meditation . . ." (Foucault, 1979:128). The mental health workers oversaw this "enclosed, segmented space, observed at every point . . . in which the slightest movements are supervised, in which all events are recorded" (Foucault 1979:128). It was their job to watch the patients and to keep a record of the fact that they were watched. Thus, as a "seclusion room," the unit kept the patients from hurting themselves or others; as a "monastery," it disciplined them and attempted to turn their attention inward.

The "time-table" of the patients was extremely spare. In fact, the APU staff talked of the inside of the unit as a place where there was (appropriately) almost nothing to do. Giuliani called this "isolation without an agenda." The notion that barrenness was useful made it a matter of pride with the staff not to "fix up" the unit's interior. One nurse explained this attitude, "We don't want to make the patients too comfortable. You play cards, watch TV, and when you get bored you make some decision where you want to go." Or, as Sam put it, "We make this *not* an alternative to life outside." The staff believed that the lack of comfort was one element that contributed to their productiveness and competence in keeping beds open; patients did not want to stay.

This aspect of the unit was something that the transient students and residents were forced to come to terms with. In this account a first-year medical student described his initial reaction to the unit and his socialization into the staff's belief in the appropriateness of the unit's austerity:

Starkness was everywhere: the loud black and white TV, the schedule of activities on the wall which no one read or followed, painted cinder-block walls . . . a bookcase without books. All the amenities for life were there, but the atmosphere was that of a prison. My sensibilities cried out for exercise, books and newspapers, real activities, daylight, and trees. When did I begin to change? . . . The "acuteness" of some patients tempered my enthusiasm for opening up the ward and providing for unmet needs. A great number of patients would not have realized the existence of different circumstances and would have exhausted all the unit's resources to the exclusion of others . . . It became clear to me that, given the restrictions of the state mental health system and the short-term nature of the unit, patients' needs would best be addressed directly and unequivocally. I came to question my original ideas of treatment. Were we there as surrogate parents with the job of providing for all of the patients' needs or were we assigned the task of attempting to turn patients around? Once I began to see it more clearly, the starkness was not as oppressive. It gained purpose and lost its former emotional content for me.

This student frames his reaction in terms of a contrast between "parenting," which would entail the provision of "exercise and trees," and "directness," the acceptance of the reality both of patients' limitations and the finitude of resources. The "questioning of original ideas" that he describes was a main theme of teaching on the unit, a process most medical students went through. Institutional barrenness took on meaning and purpose and came to be seen as an active choice rather than a deprivation.

Ben was even clearer about the congruence involved; it was an achievement rather than a failure for the unit to match the condition of the patients.

The decorations are the patients. We embellish our unit with people instead of having a static model that people can only be happy in a happy place. The starkness of the way [the patients] live [outside] is a shock; the unit is only reflecting it.

⚹ From the staff point of view, the enclosed and barren space of the back of the unit reflects the poverty and craziness of the patients, revealing them as they truly are. Removed from the everyday world, they are placed in a "holding pattern" that contrasts with the sometimes hectic pace of work in the front of the unit where the staff "engage in activities that resemble the hustle and bustle of a clearing house" (Wilson 1986:186).

〰 Part of this "hustle and bustle" resulted from the fact that the staff had a more complex relationship to the time and space of the unit than did the patients. While the patients were treated more or less alike (with the exception of seclusion or room restriction) the staff had varying degrees of control over their time and place of work, and their relationships to one another were complex and ambiguous.

In considering the relationship between the various staff members and the space of the unit, let us start with the mental health workers. The mental health workers were perceived to be (and considered themselves) in a position analogous to that of the patients.[4] They were stuck in the back of the unit, working eight-hour shifts without a private area of their own to use for breaks. Poorly paid and lacking in professional credentials, their job was to keep track of the patients, give them their meals, and call for help in case of trouble. They called themselves the "outcastes" of the unit; Trina Thorne explained that they were always trying to escape by going to the bathroom or hiding in the nurses' station. She described the best escape as "blanking out"; "I don't pay attention to the patients," she said, "unless, of course, they start to *fight*." Trina and the other mental health workers called the rest of the staff "telephone workers" who spent their time, not with the patients, but in contact with the outside world. Trina emphasized her emotional and physical distance from the other staff members, saying that she handled them "with a long-handled spoon." She and the other mental health workers refused to go to the staffing meetings at which patients were discussed, saying that "some of these people with *degrees* can't stand it if you make an intelligent remark."

These images of distance were echoed by other staff members in their descriptions of the mental health workers, whom they regarded as lazy, unreliable, and afflicted with mental problems parallel to those of the patients. One of the social workers described a mental health worker:

⚹   *He's mad because he has to work, because he's alive. He's a manic. He feels he's the one everyone dumps all the work on. He doesn't want to be here. He's been very lazy—two hour breaks, not coming back at all. When they get on him he feels he's in the right. He's being closely watched by the nursing staff for his performance.*

Even Trina, who worked with this staff member, said that when he first came to the unit "he was so much like the patients I couldn't stand it." Barbara Wilson, the nurse chairperson, believed that this similarity between the mental health workers and the patients arose from individual choices made by the workers themselves. She recounted the story of one worker who had obtained a degree and left the unit and went on to say:

> Some people just settle; they don't want to accept challenge. They are stuck by choice.

In these remarks the mental health worker is perceived to reject work, to resist discipline, and to exaggerate the amount of work. These failings are perceived to result from moral and intrapsychic weakness. Thus, like the patients, the mental health worker must be kept under surveillance; the man described above is "being watched" by the nursing staff. This man expressed his own position, angrily, as follows in an exchange with one of the nurses:

> We're just babysitters. Do you know how to change a diaper? This is what has happened to us, we have no role anymore other than catering to the patients.

"Catering to the patients" was associated with being locked up, with "babysitting," and with exclusion from the more valued and adult role of "telephone worker." The mental health workers resembled the caretakers (but not the parents) of unruly children, they also resembled both the patients themselves, and factory workers constrained by unremitting shift labor. Their position allowed the least room for movement of any on the unit.

The nurses were also shift workers who had no space of their own on the unit; however, they had more freedom of movement than the mental health workers. They chose when to go into the back of the unit and were able to direct their activity to specific patient needs, such as baths and medication. They spent much of their time in the nursing station where they were responsible for keeping records on the patients, dispensing medication, and participating in the process of matching patients to placements. All of the staff were agreed about three characteristics of the position of APU nurse. First, the job could be disturbing; it involved a particular attitude of vigilance and noninvolvement. Barbara said of the job: "Patient management is the hard part. We have psychotic, dangerous, belligerent patients; the nurses must avoid injury and be alert to volatile behavior." A new nurse was sometimes tested by being left alone with the patients. Second, the job required flexibility.

Nurses had to "be open-minded and willing to learn," according to Barbara. "Some," she said, "say they want to work with patients and then can't handle it. It takes an experienced nurse. Flexibility is important, . . . and you have to have a certain levity about [the job]."

Finally, the nurses had a higher rate of turnover than the other staff members. They had relatively good opportunities for other positions and sometimes found themselves in conflict over the nature of the job. Barbara emphasized the amount of responsibility involved:

> *There is a high chance of inexperienced nurses leaving; you have to feel OK about yourself to work with patients like these. Responsibilities involve decision making and if there are a lot of fears of violence you won't have the necessary relaxation to be unafraid.*

Sam described this in terms of the difference between what a new staff member expected and how the unit actually was:

> *A recent graduate came and wanted to save people and work in emergency settings and talk people out of doing themselves in. She discovered we were not so nice and patients weren't nice and weren't appreciative.*

Another nurse

> *always wore white and wanted to be* a nurse *but it was pathetic to see her try to reconcile role and place, always outraged, everything was wrong, the patients weren't treated right. She got into a big fight about something trivial.*

In order to stay on the unit a nurse had to accept the role of "managing" patients who weren't "treated right," she had to be flexible about the work (for example, she had to be willing to do someone else's job during periods of understaffing), and she had to find ways to "reconcile role and place."

While there was general agreement about what might make a nurse leave, the extent of the nurses' influence on the unit was a matter of dispute. Walter, for example, said that the nurses "felt all powerful" but that in fact "the mental health workers and counselors (including himself) do all the work and control the environment." Barbara, who had a relatively distanced view as a result of her administrative position, regarded the staff as unified and "on top of it" despite a "bureaucracy that does not reward you." Nancy Altman and Lillian Morgan both saw the central problem of the nursing staff as involving paperwork—that is, conflicts over who was to do specific recording chores. For Ben Caldwell, who saw the situation from a position part way outside the unit, the issue was one of "who would have power." The "system," in his view, had a built-in confusion about who was in charge of what. This Rashomon-like diversity in staff members' interpretations of the nurses' influence reflected a more general tendency on the unit: a contextualizing and relativizing of power. Although the mental workers' situation, like that of the patients, was fairly unambiguous, the "up-front" workers were enmeshed in a shifting context in which many different interpretations coexisted.

This drawing by Walter, whose desk was in the screening area, shows what the unit looked like to an "up-front" worker. He colored it to indicate the importance, to him, of different areas. The darker items at the top are the tables and chairs in the lobby, the vending machines near the guard's desk, and the bathroom. These were his areas of "solace and escape"; as an up-front, non-shift worker he was free to leave the unit and visit the lobby from time to time. The screening area and his desk (with a small X next to it) have the things "vital to doing the job," mainly the telephones and the *Diagnostic and Statistical Manual of Mental Disorders, Third Edition* (on the desk next to his). The rest of the unit, shown as small cubicles and offices drawn in an increasingly vague blue, is "least important," an area that "fades." Walter thus indicates his relative freedom of movement and his psychological distance from the "back" of the unit; for him there are others—the mental health workers and nurses—who mediate this area. His concern, like that of the other non-shift workers, is with the process of admissions (the diagnostic manual) and placement (the telephone).

For those whose relationship to the unit was less permanent, one of the central issues was its usefulness as a place for learning. For Robert Naumann, the forensic psychologist who came to the unit to help with specific patients, the unit's internal relationships were never clear; the APU, he said, "is a very slippery operation," hard to pin down. But he felt that it was a "learning ground run by the doctors *for* the doctors." The medical students and residents got lots of learning experience and good supervision; their experience was dynamic. But for the permanent staff, including himself, much less was available in terms of "learning new ways to look at things." He experienced a sense of stagnation and low morale.

Students and residents often did experience the unit as a dynamic learning ground. This drawing by a medical student indicates his view of the space of the unit as a tiered and hierarchical arrangement. The patients are an undifferentiated focal point held within a circle; at the top are the places they come from and to either side are the places to which they are "turfed." The nurses, who mediate between the patients and the residents and medical students, are not confined to a specific

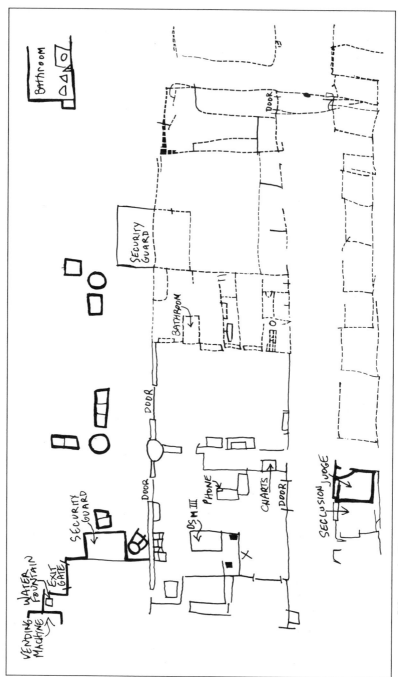

WALTER'S PERSPECTIVE

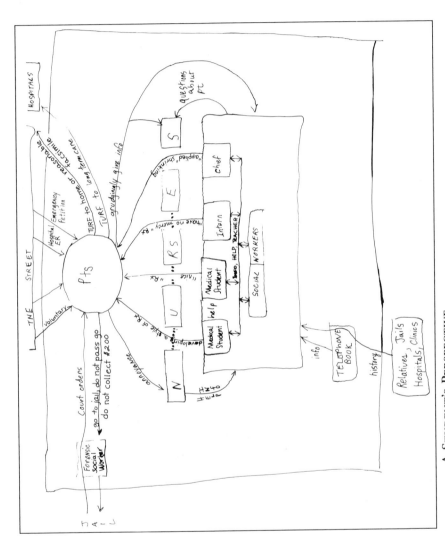

A STUDENT'S PERSPECTIVE

space. "Annoyance" from the patients passes through the nurses and is translated into "help" and "info" for the medical staff. "Questions about patients" go to the nurses; patients "grudgingly give information" to nurses and the other staff. As this student put it, "The nurses are a buffer for the doctors, and a glass wall for the patients." On the other side of the medical staff and in the same "up-front" space are the social workers, who offer "information, help, and teaching." Thus the overall space of the unit is articulated into a series of interconnected smaller spaces connected by flows of "annoyance," "help," and "information." The various kinds of relationship to patients which this student felt he was developing—"nice doctor," "applied shrinking," "developing a style of treatment," and "have no mercy"—are mediated by the nurses and backed up by the other staff.

For the residents, also, information was an important aspect of the work; they could learn from the patients and the place. Duane explained that he found the APU "not any more discouraging than anything else in medicine; you're dealing with chronic illness. The reward is that you learn a lot, because of the high turnover. Patients teach you a lot, too, because they're pros at being in hospitals." The real work, for Duane, was to make use of the apparent disadvantages of the place—its experienced patients and high turnover—to learn lessons that would serve him well in future professional work.

Thus the attention to the front of the unit expressed in Walter's drawing was characteristic of the higher paid, more professional members of the unit's staff. Status was correlated with mobility, privacy, and distance from the patients. The psychiatrists had the greatest degree of control over space and time, working part-time out of private offices. Their orientation was to the smooth functioning of the unit as a whole; Ben believed, and had conveyed to Sam, that it was their task to "take care of the staff as if they were patients." He considered democracy incompatible with the unit's style while at the same time providing an atmosphere of pragmatic problem solving oriented to the patients. Barbara described Ben as having "a unique way of supervising. He gives you room to go; if you've made a mess he'll say, 'Let's not look at the problem but look at the solution.'" Sam spoke of the mixture of freedom and constraint implied by this style:

> *Things here are done in a very authoritarian manner, like pre-revolutionary Russia. Ben is the Tsar, but he is removed and he gives sanction to me. But there are certain limits to my power in style and substance. You can do whatever you want with patients but you have to maintain a consistent style with staff. If you had sensitivity groups and reacted to staff discontent you'd open a can of worms. The place works by not responding to staff complaints and aspirations.*

The more powerful staff members tried to ignore the "stuck" feelings expressed by those less powerful. Sam recognized that the staff, like the patients, longed to move on to somewhere less restricted, but he admitted that few had the power to do so; "Everyone here is looking for something else; the MDs expect to find it but the others know they won't."

A counterpoint to this attitude toward the rest of the staff (and to the notion that their feelings were a "can of worms") was the psychiatrists' belief that the unit was partially hidden from the outside world, especially the administration. Administrators, in their view, could not "handle or understand" the unit and had to be protected from some of its methods of operation. The administration cooperated in protecting itself through what the psychiatrists called "active ignorance." Thus a precarious balance between visibility and invisibility characterized the unit's relationship to the outside, with the psychiatrists acting as a buffer for the rest of the staff. This hiddenness of the unit, its position in the unconscious of psychiatry, was related to the issue of efficient disposition, for the staff accomplished their work in part through the violation of strict role and paperwork requirements. As Sam said, sardonically, of his and Ben's relationship to the outside, "One of us has to be here all the time to keep out the do-gooders."

IV

This is like the TV program "Taxi." All we have is the dispatching station and each other.

—SAM WISHINSKI

The staff of the APU were engaged in the sort of activity Goffman called "people-work." In his classic account of the mental hospital of the 1950s, Goffman pointed out that the people who enter an institution as inmates become "objects and products" of the work of the staff. This objectification is often highly ritualized, while at the same time being contradicted by the constant emergence of subjectivity and the possibility of sympathy (1961).[5]

Several recent studies describe the "special requirements" (to use Goffman's terminology) of handling people as objects when the main objective is to "place," "dispose of," "dispatch," or "turf" patients by moving them on to another location. In *Disposable Patients* Matthews (1980) describes a psychiatric emergency room in a general hospital where residents learn to minimize their work by "dumping" patients onto other services, avoiding patients, or redefining patients' problems as "non-emergent." In this context a resident's skill consists in his ability to "sell" patients to other facilities and to conduct interviews and other screening procedures with dispatch. A similar orientation is discussed by Wilson, who describes emergency psychiatry work as a "dispatching process" in which the staff experience "an intensely felt time pressure that derives from a number of sources, including legal mandates . . . and the influx of new admissions constantly lining up for the limited bed space" (1986:184). She suggests that such facilities exist in a contradictory "ideological context that simultaneously advocates administrative efficiency and medical model theory and treatment," despite the limited resources for dispersing patients back into the community.

That this kind of pressure and conflict is not unique to psychiatry is suggested by Mizrahi in *Getting Rid of Patients,* which describes the work of medical residents in a large public hospital. They too find themselves "swamped" with admissions in the face of a shortage of beds; the issue of beds, Mizrahi says, "was a major preoccupation of house staff involved in admitting and receiving patients" (1986:48). Residents evolved numerous strategies for getting rid of patients, including various means of speeding up hospitalization and complex maneuvers to transfer patients to others or prevent them from getting in. Patients, according to Mizrahi, were "objectified and discounted" as a result of this strategizing, whereas the staff developed a cynically instrumental attitude toward their work.

The situation of the APU resembles those described in these accounts; it is a public institution that accepts those who cannot go elsewhere (for reasons of behavior, insurance, or chronicity), thereby committing itself to serve far more people than it has room for. The APU staff developed a strategic and instrumental orientation to their work, treating patients, in many cases, primarily as "disposition problems." The work of Matthews and Mizrahi suggests that this form of objectification differs from that described by Goffman, because the issue is no longer the management of a relatively stable population of chronic patients, but rather the management of *movement.* ⌐APU

From the perspective of the APU staff, one source of efficiency in the management of movement is the unit's capacity to merge the "form" and the "content" of the treatment of patients. The form of the unit is its existence as an enclosure, a space of confinement, from which it is impossible to escape. The staff are explicit about the prison-like character of this space; they also make clear that its discipline consists, first, in the ordered arrangement of the space of the patients, a space in which they are distributed and watched, and, second, in the monotonous regularity of the patients' days. This space is stark, providing no activities. But it is this very starkness that makes the space useful and thus becomes its content as well as its form. It is a "holding environment" for those too disturbed to remain outside, and its efficiency rests in the provision of "isolation without an agenda"; patients are both soothed by such a place and (presumably or hopefully) motivated to leave it. Thus, as Dreyfus and Rabinow put it, "The goal desired and the techniques designed to achieve it merge" (1983).

This merging occurs at the level of the staff as well. The situation of the patients is markedly different from that of the staff in many ways, and the staff often see the patients as wholly other. But they also see themselves "stuck" in the same space so that throughout the staff hierarchy we find images of watching and being watched. Thus the mental health workers are described as "like the patients" by a social worker, the staff as a whole are "like the patients" to the psychiatrists, and the psychiatrists in turn consider themselves both visible and invisible to the administration. They are "supervisors perpetually supervised" (Foucault 1979) who also search for "solace." *everybody being watched*

Thus the staff regard their space as a site both of discipline and of ambiguity and escape. The proper way to escape is through moral effort, an internal alignment of one's goals with the possibility of improving one's status, as is implied in the descriptions of the mental health workers as "lazy" and "stuck by choice." But there are many other escapes—temporary, precarious, and inherent in the same disciplinary space that seems, from one angle, so encompassing. There is the bathroom, the lounge, the absence from work, the refuge that can be found in "relaxation." The staff both admire the enclosed and inescapable quality of their workspace and look for its margins; Ben's comment that the patients could be happy in an unhappy place extended to an insistence on the staff's potential for resistance and humor. The staff seem at once to recognize the need to order the space so that it has no margins and edges and to look for these margins and use them.[6]

This use of the margins is related to the ways the staff describe their power or lack of it. The official hierarchy provides several distinct lines of command, while at the same time the staff describe their experience in a network of ambiguous and shifting influences.[7] No one agrees on who "has" power, describing instead "innumerable points of confrontation" (Foucault 1980) in which there is an emphasis on relationship and context. Thus Walter can say that the mental health workers have power (because they deal with the patients), whereas they describe themselves as powerless at the hands of the "telephone workers." Despite (or perhaps because) of the shifting nature of power on the unit, the staff exhibited cohesion in much of their everyday interaction; this cohesion was centered on the task of patient disposition and resulted from agreement as to the nature of the work.

TWO

We Discharge in Ten Days

I

If Jesus came in we'd lock him up.

—STAFF SAYING[1]

Working here is like being in front of an accident.

—ANTHONY GIULIANI

Marilyn Nolan became violent and disruptive on a bus headed from New York to Midway City. She was brought by the police to the APU, where she allowed herself to be admitted voluntarily. A quiet, neat, middle-aged woman with an unassuming demeanor, Nolan spent most of her time in her room. When she did emerge, she sat stiffly in the day room, staring at a plastic-encased picture of Jesus which she carried everywhere she went. Some detective work on the part of the staff revealed that she had a doctor and social worker in New York and had been in a group home there, after many years of intermittent hospitalization. She wanted to return to New York, though not to the group home. As a voluntary patient she could not be kept or medicated against her will, so her treatment became a race against her symptoms: would her welfare check arrive in time, allowing her to take the bus back to New York before, as Sam said, "she gets crazy again"? Here "crazy" meant "so violent they won't allow her on a bus," for Nolan remained delusional despite her calm behavior. She believed she was God. Sam talked to her and tried to prepare her for the bus trip back to New York:

SAM: I've heard you've had more messages from God?

NOLAN: I *am* God, along with God the Father and the Holy Spirit. If I don't leave . . .

SAM: . . . will I fry?

NOLAN: It's not funny! I'm sure you don't think it's funny.

SAM: Will your being God interfere with your using the transport system?

NOLAN: No.

SAM: It's sort of a comedown for God to take Trailways.

NOLAN: I'd rather take Amtrak but unfortunately the fascists have taken it over.

SAM: If you tell people you are God you will get shipped back to a mental hospital.

NOLAN: But if I can't cash a check, I will have to tell the bank officials I am God.

SAM: I predict you will then be shipped off to the looney bin.

NOLAN [without sarcasm]: Thank you for your advice.

In the meantime, the staff played a cat-and-mouse game with their counterparts in New York. Nolan was discussed at a staff meeting.

SOCIAL WORKER: The lady in New York says we're discharging her on short notice.

SAM: *She* thinks it's short notice! Now my idea would be to call the doctor there *after* she's on the bus. They will dilly dally until we do something. We can write in the aftercare note: "Appointment made with Doctor X." She's a voluntary patient and we can argue that we have to let her go and that the people up there can decide they won't meet her. The brother here in Midway City may be a resource. Let's knock on all these doors and see which one opens.

Finally the social workers alerted their contacts in New York, made the short trip downtown, and put Nolan on a bus. Later a call came from the social worker in New York. Nolan had disappeared; she never got off the bus. At the next meeting she was discussed again:

SAM: Write a progress note about this and call Trailways and the minister.

SOCIAL WORKER: I'm the last to see her.

LILLIAN: That's why we put them on the bus and say "Bye-bye." Good thing she didn't take Amtrak.

SAM: Her secret agenda was probably to get admitted to Bellevue. We can call and ask if they have God. They'll say, "Which one?"

Three aspects of Nolan's case were typical of the APU. The first was the difficulty of her situation, the second was the way the staff concentrated on getting her out, and the third was the ambiguous ending of the story. No one ever found out what happened to her, though she lingered in the memory of the staff as "God who took Trailways."

Nolan was in an extreme situation: penniless, psychotic, and friendless in a strange city. The unit's patients were often in trouble of this magnitude; when Nolan was on the unit, the seven or eight patients there with her had equally difficult situations. These excerpts from patients' charts convey a little of the sheer enormity of their problems.

■   The patient is a 34-year-old black male here on an emergency petition [used for involuntary hospitalization in emergencies] for bizarre behavior. He has a history of hospitalization at the state facility. He is delusional and thinks he has been swallowing snakes. He was hallucinating, agitated, and suicidal at admission and was placed in seclusion, where he was in a daze and spent his time picking at the walls.

■   A new patient has come in on court order [for evaluation after arrest]. He was playing with his feces in his jail cell. He claims he is a doctor, responsible for the welfare of the world. He can't give his social security number or any other information and the name he has given doesn't seem to be his own.

■   The police found this patient walking down the street naked. They took him to the University Emergency Room, which sent him to the APU as "John Doe." The unit's staff tracked down his family, who said that he had become violent after taking PCP [a street drug]; they had locked him in a bathroom, from which he had escaped by breaking down a wall.

How did the APU staff think about these patients? First, it is important to note that these are typical emergency admissions and were therefore considered by the staff to be precisely those patients who belonged on the APU. Later we will consider examples of patients who were not "emergencies" but who still had to be accommodated by the unit.

It is in the nature of emergencies that they are not the stuff of reflection. The APU staff dealt immediately and directly with acutely disturbed patients, medicating them, secluding them if necessary, and getting to work quickly on the task of getting them out. They spoke directly to the patients, as Sam does to Nolan, of the implications of their behavior and of the consequences of being in or getting out of the "looney bin." To one another they spoke casually of the patients' condition: patients were "impossible," "crazy," "loose," "nuts," "out to lunch," and "bananas." Patients "climbed the walls" and a primary task on the unit was to "get them off the walls."

Although the staff were concerned with distinguishing psychotic from criminal behavior and both from physical illness, they recognized a kind of bedrock of "craziness" that required no justification for intervention. The staff would agree with Ingleby that "it has to be admitted that . . . there remains a residue in most 'mental illnesses' which is refractory to all ordinary procedures of understanding and empathy" (1980:60).[2] Playing with feces, undressing in the street, insisting one is God: although encounters with such behavior were commonplace for the APU staff, the behavior itself had a refractory residue of incoherence that defined the otherness of the patients and made their confinement appear logical and inevitable.

This day to day, pragmatic relationship to the patients' craziness rested on certain assumptions that were basic to the everyday work of the unit, though they might be questioned in moments of reflection. One was the necessity for control inherent in emergency work. When the staff reflected on the implications of emergency work, they pointed out that an emergency has two components. One is the "emergent" behavior, behavior that is disruptive and dangerous to the patient or to others. Such behavior, in their view, necessitates and justifies a social reaction of control and isolation. The other component is the social context of the behavior and, especially, the conditions that make it intolerable to the patient or those around him. As one writer on psychiatric emergencies puts it:

> The psychiatric emergency does not exist until it is placed within a social setting. For example, suicidal ideation not brought to the attention of others . . . is never identified as an emergency. Once the elements of a patient's stress or danger are brought into the social system, however, the evaluation and disposition process grind on until the stress and danger are reduced or eliminated. (Cumming 1983:7)[3]

The staff recognized that pressure for intervention is not simply a function of the craziness of the behavior and that one person's emergency might be another's daily life. Sometimes, for example, an over-eager student might be reminded that a condition that seemed intolerable to her might be "the patient's highest level of functioning in years." However, the staff knew that their job was the management of intolerable situations and in general they left the sorting out of the question "intolerable to whom?" until after the situation itself was under control.

This understanding that emergencies inevitably combined treatment with the more obvious forms of social control had implications for the way the staff saw their work. One Douglass Center psychiatrist, speaking formally to a group of residents, explained that emergency workers had a "societally defined responsibility" for "social control." "Managing difficult patients," he said, "challenges all of our learned behaviors and personal ethics and our stated and unstated societal norms." In a "behavioral emergency" society expects fast action without providing clear expectations. On the APU, the "learned behaviors" of caretakers—especially their resistance to direct coercion of other people—contradicted the kind of action required to "manage difficult patients."

The assumption that illness was "inside" the patient complemented this view of emergencies. Diagnosis on the APU will be considered in chapter 5. In the most general sense, however, the test of whether someone belonged on the unit was whether his emergent behavior could be translated into a psychiatric (rather than medical or legal) problem category. Most patients admitted to the unit were diagnosed with serious psychiatric illness such as schizophrenia, manic depressive illness, psychotic depression, or borderline personality disorder. Many had long histories of psychiatric illness and hospitalization. Some patients were suicidal, or had harmed or threatened someone; many had drug or alcohol problems. Many patients, like Nolan, lived with apparently permanent delusions that seriously distorted their perceptions; others suffered acute episodes of psychosis interspersed with periods of relatively normal functioning. Most of the time these problems appeared to the staff to be inside the patients, both the manifestation and the definition of their condition; the staff would speak of "his" manic depression and "her" schizophrenia.

The disorientation, hallucinations, delusions, or mood disturbances that brought patients to the hospital could often be relieved with medications such as haloperidol (Haldol), fluphenazine (Prolixin), thioridizine (Mellaril), antidepressants, and lithium. These medications affect the severe symptoms of psychosis.[4] They were the main treatment the unit had to offer for most patients, a way to alleviate symptoms so that the patient could either return to his previous situation or move on to treatment at a longer-term facility. Seclusion (that is, locking patients into a bare room devoid of furniture, where they were checked frequently to make sure they didn't hurt themselves) was sometimes used while staff waited for the medication to take effect. Some patients were calmed by the medicine, but remained psychotic; others "cleared" and within hours of admission could talk to staff about what had happened to them and where they wanted to go. In this use of medication and isolation the staff, as one psychiatrist put it, treated "behavior as a clinical entity in itself." Their main interest was in changing the patients' behavior enough so that they could go elsewhere.

Improvement as a result of medication was not a simple thing. For many patients medication had little effect on the deep disturbances in thinking and behavior that had brought them to the hospital. Other patients experienced dramatic changes as a result of medication but were not able or willing to continue taking it once they left the hospital. For most patients, the medicine did little to relieve the conditions of life that were the context of their disturbed mental condition. Patients' "episodes" of illness and "breaks" into psychosis had as their background less acute but more pervasive forms of distress.

I gathered information on all the admissions to the APU over a three-month period that reveals something of the background of the patients (ninety-seven patients). Almost 80 percent of the unit's patients had been hospitalized before, either at the Douglass Center (40 percent) or at another facility. Approximately 80 percent were unemployed. Some lived on disability payments in boarding houses or single room hotels or missions, often under wretched conditions. Over 10 percent were officially considered "at large" or homeless; others had an address (because they gave addresses of friends or relatives) but were, in fact, without a reliable place to live. Others lived in families with difficult or abusive relationships. About a third of the patients were "court-ordered," which meant that they had been arrested, sometimes on petty charges such as vagrancy and trespassing, and were to be assessed as to whether they belonged in the criminal justice or the mental health system. Another third were "certified," that is, admitted involuntarily for a brief period because of their disruptive or destructive behavior. The APU admitted more men (70 percent) than women and more blacks (65 percent) than whites; most patients were between the ages of twenty and fifty.

Ben and Sam were referring to the magnitude of the patients' problems and their relationship to the social and economic problems of the city when they told me that the APU was the unconscious of psychiatry. These problems were of everyday, overwhelming visibility on the unit; patients came in hungry, dirty, and lice-ridden, and complained directly of a lack of money, housing, and social support. At the level of day to day encounter the "starkness" of patients' lives could not be avoided and was recognized to be inseparable from their symptoms. Lillian told her social work students that they could "expect to get their fingers dirty" working in a place like the APU. The staff, especially the social work staff, worked to deal with the patients' problems at the level of job and apartment hunting, the welfare system, looking for relatives, or otherwise trying to affect their living situations.

At the same time, the environment from which patients came was a kind of "background noise" that the staff noticed to a greater or lesser degree depending on the situation. In reflective moments, the staff sometimes saw the unit's surroundings as a "jungle" in which anyone might become deranged. Rarely, however, did staff members speculate directly about economic or political causes of the patients' problems.[5] They were able to tune out the larger social background in part because their notions of illness and emergency enabled them to place the difficulties of patients in the context of proximate internal and social disorder. But perhaps more importantly, the necessity for direct action on one pressing problem after another involved the staff with the complex field of give and take that constituted the unit's "options for disposition." The process of disposition had a fascination and immediacy and held out a possibility of success compared with which speculation about larger causes of the patients' troubles seemed futile and discouraging.

II

We discharge in ten days so that we won't be tempted to treat them and screw up.

—BEN CALDWELL

. . . it is something strictly American to conceive a space that is filled always filled with moving.

—GERTRUDE STEIN, quoted in Harvey (1985:16)

Nolan was discharged from the APU within a week of admission. It is apparent from the conversation about her that the staff regarded their speed of operations as exceptional compared to that of other facilities (thus, Sam says of the social worker in New York, "*She* thinks it's short notice") and that their object in connecting with the patients' previous caretakers was to get them to take the patient back, even if this required some trickery ("My idea would be to call the doctor *after* we put her on the bus"). The staff assumed that a patient like Nolan was a problem to anyone responsible for her and they were proud that they knew how to move her on without dawdling like their counterparts. They were motivated by their desire to maintain empty beds, by their recognition that they had "little to offer her" in the way of treatment, and by the fact that they could not keep her against her will. At the same time they were constrained by an awareness of their responsibility for her safety; this is the reason for the stress on documentation and for their care in placing her, bodily, on the bus.

We saw that the staff described the unit as an enclosed and prison-like space. They also used images that referred to its being a "space always filled with moving." Sam explained that the unit was like the "bedroom on a submarine" with 150 to 200 patients cycling through in the same way that the crew of a submarine sleeps in shifts.[6] Robert Naumann described the unit as a whirlpool that sucked patients in, quickly sifted them, and ejected them to other parts of the river. A medical student said that the unit was like a bus station: "If you don't see results (with the patients) you don't have to keep them, just dump them someplace else." Ben Caldwell, who was the original architect of this attitude, explained:

The idea that the patient belongs in the hospital leads to slow discharge. Here, everyone is an inappropriate admission. I don't admit patients, I discharge them.

The staff had to start thinking about discharge as soon as a patient came in. From the beginning, Ben said:

We aim toward separation. Other wards have an orientation for new patients. It would be absurd to "orient" someone to the APU. Do you get an orientation when you go to a hotel?

Patients didn't need orientation because their stays on the unit were so brief and because the unit's simplicity gave little to orient them to. In this drawing, Walter shows the unit as a funnel through which patients must "keep moving, no stopping" on their way to the bus station. (Nolan was by no means the only patient to enter and/or leave the unit via the bus station).[7]

The unit maintained a network of relationships to other units, facilities, and agencies. This network was not reducible to a "map" of possible dispositions but was fluid and contingent; Ben explained it by saying, "We have a protoplasmic style." When I tried to talk him into drawing me a map of the unit's "environment" he refused. The space I was asking him to draw was, he said, four-dimensional and not amenable to representation on paper. It was rather like shopping in an old-fashioned farmer's market. My path through the market, and my negotiations with different sellers, will differ from yours; my path and negotiations will even vary from one shopping trip to the next. As the active agent in putting together my dinner, I am the "converting influence" between the merchants.[8] The staff, in other words, experienced their relationships to disposition as a movement among individually negotiated options. Ben said it was "like trying to carry jello without a bowl."

This drawing by Lillian shows the patient (client)[9] entering the unit, either through emergency services or the forensic clinic, and becoming

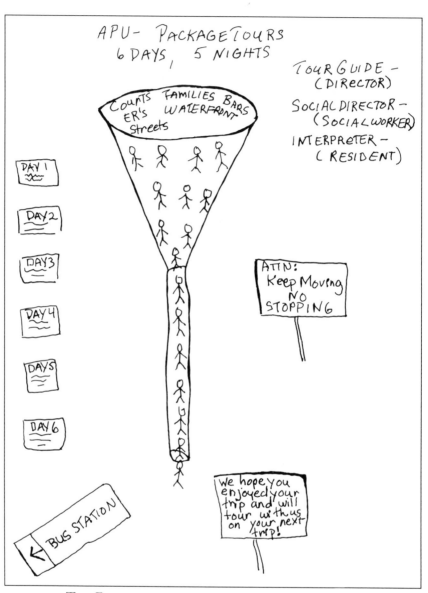

The Funnel

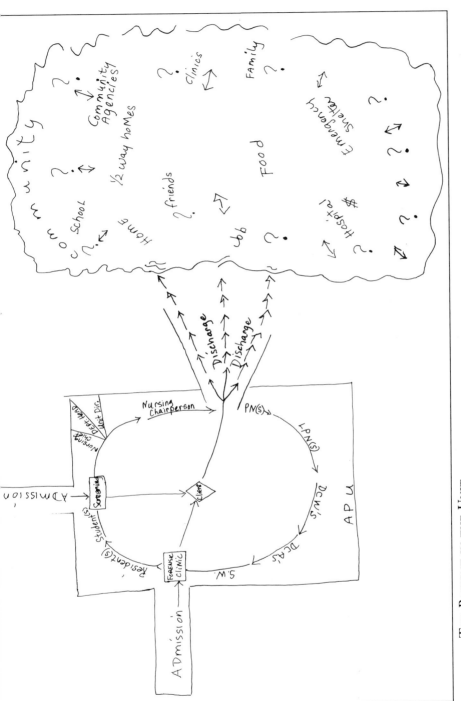

THE PATIENT IN THE UNIT

the center of a circle of attention from nurses, social workers, direct care workers, and residents. The inside of the unit is pictured as enclosed, orderly, and focused. Discharge is represented by vigorously drawn arrows, as though the patient is tumbling out of a chute. The outside world resembles Ben's "bowl of jello." Ringed by a dim, wavy line representing "community" are many question marks and two-way arrows in a space of unconnected "resources"; "food," "friends," "community agencies," "family," and "emergency shelter" float together, undifferentiated and disordered.

This was the view of the person on the unit who had the most experience and skill in placing patients. Robert Naumann, also very experienced, echoed it when he said of his work with the criminal justice system:

> Sometimes I feel like I'm a detective; I'm working on this giant jigsaw puzzle and I don't know whether I can get all the pieces together.

These staff members, along with Ben Caldwell, Walter Boyd, and other long-term workers, had developed an actor-centered perspective on the outside world. They saw it as a shifting field in which decisions could be made only as *particular* staff members, patients, and outside agencies intersected. This intersection was often framed in terms of "deviousness and indirection," the kind of strategy that enabled Sam to get Cunningham onto a ward upstairs or that made Nolan's case an exercise in the manipulation of the mental health workers in New York. But deviousness had to be balanced with concern for reputation—not the reputation of the unit as a whole but reputation as an individual. Lillian, especially, was concerned that agencies she worked with all the time trust her so that she could turn to them repeatedly for help. Contrasting the unit with the rest of the hospital, she explained that maintaining possibilities for disposition had to be a constant concern.

> It's just a different world down here. Our objective is to have beds empty . . . The stress [on APU workers] is when there are no beds in the hospital—can the patient go? It's always you . . . on the line . . . Turfing depends on your reputation. You tell *people [outside about a patient]* "*He's a real zero, but we think you can handle it.*"

A social work student drew this picture of the way the unit worked. The most orderly of the images I collected, it shows the unit as a passageway organized into stages of treatment and the outside world as sets of possible "referrals" and destinations. At the top the student shows the various ways patients came to the hospital—in crisis, brought in by families concerned with their behavior, referred by the "community,"

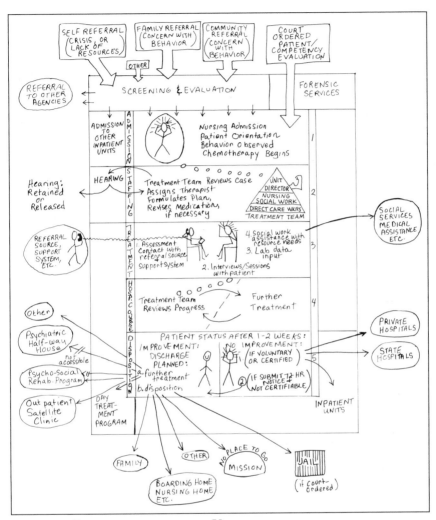

Passage through the Unit

or ordered by the court. Court-ordered patients were admitted through the forensic psychologist, whereas others came in through screening and evaluation. Once on the unit, the patient (seen tearing his/her hair) was evaluated and given medication. Note that this student suggests the existence of the "patient orientation" whose absence Ben is proud of. (I suspect that she had not actually observed the orientation of patients—so far as I know they were simply shown to their rooms—but had seen it referred to in a written protocol.) The patient was discussed in a staffing meeting (a biweekly meeting of the unit's staff) and assigned a treatment team consisting of a resident or medical student, nurse, and social worker. These staff members concentrated on linking the patient to the outside world (social services, support system); the staff member, faced with the patient still tearing his hair, is simultaneously writing in a notebook and talking on the telephone. After further treatment, two possibilities are shown: discharge to outpatient care if improved, or discharge to other hospital facilities if not improved.

The lower section of this drawing points to the major division between dispositions: some dispositions depended on a patient's ability to function independently, whereas others provided continued inpatient care. An important consideration in deciding between them is indicated by "hearing," "jail," and the arrow that points from "not certifiable" to the "discharge planned" category. The unit was linked to the legal system, both by its management of court-ordered patients and by the requirement that patients' rights be considered in decisions about treatment.

In the sections that follow, I am concerned to show how these "options for disposition" appeared to the staff of the APU. The student's drawing will serve as an organizing device, but it is important to remember Ben's metaphors of the market and the jello without a bowl. Disposition was an uncertain and ad hoc process that belied the social welfare terminology used in the drawing; "social services," "referral," "community," and "treatment options" were part of a sanitized vocabulary that obscured the reality of what Lillian—"point-blank" as always—called turfing.[10]

HOSPITALS

The Douglass Center functioned as a short-term psychiatric hospital; on most of its wards patients stayed from three to five months, a period in sharp contrast to the years patients used to spend in large, rural state hospitals. The APU was the smallest of these wards and had the shortest patient stays. The nature of its function in the hospital depended on one's point of view. If the emphasis was on "how patients get into the hospital" the APU could be considered part of the "emergency services" that fed patients onto the hospital's longer-term wards. Thus Walter Boyd said, "We're the mouth that feeds the body"—the entry place for patients who later moved onto other hospital wards. On the other hand, if the emphasis was on "how patients are kept out of the hospital" the APU could be seen as part of the hospital's "screening" mechanism—it functioned to "weed out" (Lillian) patients who proved after a week or two of treatment that they did not need to enter a longer-term ward.

Ben graphically phrased this perspective in a metaphor of infection: "I think of screening as protecting the APU. Only when the bacteria become virulent and invasive do we have to call on the APU to neutralize the unwelcome invaders." The APU was successful when it disposed of its "unwelcome invaders"—[the patients!]—outside the hospital.

Which of these images was primary depended in large part on whether beds were available in the hospital. Sometimes the APU staff found it quite easy to "send a patient upstairs" to another hospital ward, and they often did so when a patient's condition did not change and long-term care was clearly indicated. Sometimes, when the hospital was full or the patient was "undesirable," it was difficult to convince "the people upstairs" to open one of their beds to an APU patient. Thus the unit's relationship to the upstairs was ambivalent and unstable. One nurse who had worked at the state hospital commented that she found it unusual that "the units [at the Douglass Center] are all so separate." She didn't know anyone "upstairs" and noted that the staff only carried keys to their own units, reinforcing a sense of isolation. The other units in the hospital "manipulated out of" taking patients they didn't want and, in her view, thought of the APU as a "dump." Walter Boyd said that the APU was a "mystery" to others in the building, a place that operated under different rules and assumptions than the longer-term units.

When the "upstairs" could or would not accept a patient who needed hospitalization, the APU staff had to turn to other hospitals in the area. Their options were limited. Patients with insurance who came into screening were referred to private hospitals; the Douglass Center, as Sam put it, "defended its beds for the indigent." The most likely placement for APU patients who had no insurance was what the staff called the "chronic hospital," meaning the state hospital that accepted patients on a long-term basis. But as a result of deinstitutionalization, beds at long-term state facilities were limited; patients had to "qualify" as "unable to live in the community" and even then there was often a wait for a bed. Both patients and staff sometimes saw the state hospital in a rather nostalgic light, as a place where patients could be fully dependent without pressure to leave. Faced with patients who wanted to be in the hospital but did not "qualify" as sick enough, the staff sometimes talked wistfully of the "old days when they had farms" and patients were not expected to "function" outside the hospital.

Two kinds of hospital placements were relatively easy to make. Midway City was divided into catchment areas, each with its own public hospital and mental health facilities. New patients' addresses were checked to make sure they were in the right catchment area; if not, they could be transferred into the hands of those responsible for their own area. Similarly, the staff tried to find out whether a new patient was a veteran and could be sent to the VA hospital.

THE COURTS

The APU had intimate ties with the legal system, which the staff usually referred to by the general term "the courts." One function of the unit was the evaluation of "court-ordered" patients. These patients had either been ordered "evaluated for competency to stand trial" or had been "sent from jail" because of their bizarre behavior. Robert Naumann, the forensic psychologist, was charged with the interface between the legal system and the hospital and with seeing court-ordered patients through their hospital stay. These patients made up about 30 percent of APU patients.

The interface of the hospital and the court system was intricate and sometimes awkward. Some patients were arrested on trivial charges such as "vagrancy" or "littering"; once in jail, they were sent to the APU for evaluation. Often, the solution was to "drop charges" and keep the patient in the hospital. Other patients were sent for evaluation for more serious offenses. The APU staff was expected to determine whether or not the patient was able to understand the procedures involved in a trial. But, as Robert Naumann said, "Insanity is a legal definition; there is nothing in psychiatry that corresponds to it. 'Psychotic' is different." For example, he said, a person who has stopped taking medication ("voluntarily") is legally responsible for his or her behavior if the person later becomes psychotic. Naumann's job was to translate between the two systems, trying, in each case, to find an outcome acceptable to both.

> *I go over the options [for court-ordered patients] with the APU staff. Then I go and do the same thing with the people at the courts and I talk it over and negotiate. It is less important to know and remember everything and more important to know where to find things [out]. I see that as my principal job.*

The issues were clear-cut in cases of patients who could be easily assigned to one or the other category—either clearly psychotic (in which case the charges could be dropped) or clearly not insane (in which case they were returned to jail). But in more ambiguous cases the APU and the courts (and police) were involved in parallel practices of turfing. As Ben put it, "The police officer is doing the same thing we are—moving the person along." In these cases decisions about which system a patient belonged in were often contingent on the immediate situation on the unit. For example:

■ A patient has been given a medical test that turned out to be invalid. He is on court-order. Sam tells the resident that if the unit was full they would tell the court that they couldn't keep him. But since the census is low, they can do the test again. Sam explains, "This is not too clear-cut. . . . the court would like him here, instead of in jail or out on bail."

When the staff felt that a patient did not belong on the unit, they could be adept at determining "competency."

■ Duane Powers and a medical student conduct an interview with a court-ordered patient who is being evaluated for competency after cashing a check she found on the street. Duane tries to assess her knowledge of the courts ["Are there firemen who shout 'you're guilty'"?] and she inadvertently reveals that she does understand how the courts work [that there is a judge, jury, etc.]. Once she sees she's been trapped she tries to back down ["What are you talking about?"] but it's too late. After she leaves Duane says, "Now that's what you might call an *applied* psychiatric interview! It's not in the books, but . . ."

Another aspect of the legal system was the hearing. Patients who were admitted involuntarily were entitled to a hearing to determine whether they could be retained against their will (that is, whether they were "dangerous to self or others").[11] These were held once a week in the hospital by a hearing officer and a public defender. The patient was usually accompanied by the psychiatrist assigned to his case. The psychiatrist read from the patient's chart and explained why the patient should be retained, whereas the defender tried to use the information at hand to argue on the patient's behalf. Patients who were not retained could not be held against their will; thus, in the social work student's drawing, the patient who is not "certifiable" (that is, has been involuntarily admitted but cannot be legally retained) is entitled to leave regardless of "improvement." This was the situation with Nolan; the staff could not legally keep her against her will even though they regarded her as crazy. They wanted to get her out and back to New York before she became too deranged to make the trip.[12]

The staff were aware that they walked a fine line between keeping patients against their will and letting them go when they might be dangerous to themselves and others. On the one hand, the hearing and commitment process and the rules against involuntary medication limited their ability to keep patients like Nolan; on the other hand, they could be held responsible if they released a patient who later committed a crime.

REHABILITATION AND OUTPATIENT FACILITIES

As the social worker shows in her drawing, an "improved" patient could (in theory) go to "further treatment" in an outpatient clinic, a halfway house, or a rehabilitation program. Five outpatient clinics were linked to the Douglass Center, each serving a particular neighborhood within the larger area served by the center. These clinics provided medication, counseling and community services; by far the greatest portion of the catchment area's psychiatric patients were served, not by the hospital, but by these clinics. When clinic patients had to be hospitalized, they were sent to the Douglass Center. The outpatient director of the hospital who oversaw the clinics said: "It's a battlefield out there and we send our casualties to the APU." The "casualties" were those patients who became psychotic and/or unable to manage any longer on their own.

Patients were discharged from the APU with a referral for "aftercare" to the clinic; an appointment was set up before the patient left the hospital. It was these appointments, which patients often did not keep, that constituted one aspect of the administration's "aftercare" problem.[13] For Lillian, who made many of these appointments, it was the possibility of aftercare that made the quick discharge of a patient tolerable. She said, "It's when aftercare fouls up that I feel frustrated, when the clinics change medications, or an appointment isn't kept. Patients become chronic when they get better inpatient than outpatient care." But for most of the APU staff outpatient aftercare was something of an abstraction. They documented that they had "referred" the patients they discharged, but they did not "follow up" on patients after they left. In fact, it was not clear precisely how this could be done, given the pressure of incoming patients and the confused circumstances to which many patients were discharged.

In her drawing the social worker student blocked off the lines leading to "rehab" and "halfway houses" because these were merely theoretical options. In reality, such placements either were not available to Douglass Center patients or were not accessible to patients without insurance.

An "improved" patient could be discharged to family, if one was available. Many patients on the APU did not have families or had families who were unwilling to take them. When no immediate family was in evidence, the staff questioned patients to try to find more distant relatives who might be willing to take the patient in. As Sam put it, "At a middle-class hospital the staff are always trying to find other than family placement. They talk about parentectomy. Here it's such a thrill when the family wants the patient."

Missions (homeless shelters) were also considered an option for discharge by the APU staff, who believed that they were the only choice some patients had. As Naumann put it, "As long as someone's reasonably provided for and inflicting no damage, are we right to insist on things like a regular place to live? Sometimes all the patient wants . . . is discharge to a mission. Lots of other things have been tried and not worked out." [14]

Boarding homes were another possibility for patients who could manage somewhat independently. These were run by private citizens who charged patients whatever they received in disability or welfare payments. These homes were appreciated by the APU staff as a last resort for patients who had nowhere else to go, and they had the advantage that the boarding home owner might take an interest in the patient. [15] The most difficult patients to place were those who, in the common expression of the staff, had burned their bridges, and for these the boarding homes were the last step before the mission. The staff knew that boarding home owners would quickly eject a disruptive patient. For example, a resident said of an alcoholic patient, "I'll just give him one shot at a group home and after that it's the mission." Lillian, describing a patient for whom "the only place was a group home," explained that she told him "You have burned everything. I can't offer you anything."

In a conversation about a patient newly admitted from court, Duane and Sam discussed the dwindling of resources for a patient. As in many such conversations on the unit, the question of "responsibility" dangles, shifting back and forth between the patient, who has been ejected from a home and arrested, and the lack of places available to him.

DUANE: I just interviewed the new guy. We'll probably drop charges and send him to the mission if he can't remember his sister's address. He was just released from the boarding home and was on the street for a few days until he started directing traffic.

SAM: Hopefully he was undermedicated and medicating him up will . . .

DUANE: Like Lillian said, he might have been trying to get back into the hospital . . . he's not so bad right now.

SAM: His best disposition [the boarding home] is down the drain and there's so little to turn to.

DUANE: Too bad these rooming houses are drying up . . .

This image of the drying up of a resource suggests the APU view of the world of dispositions as a landscape shaped by what often seemed to be forces of nature. Like the social circumstances of patients' lives, the social causes and ramifications of the lack of resources—the lessening of government support, the changing character of neighborhoods where housing had become expensive, new forms of custodial care—constituted background noise. As with the patients themselves, the problem for the staff was not explanation but action—how to make the most of the little that was available.

THE UNIVERSITY

An important part of the outside world was the University, a major medical school ten blocks away from the mental health center. In the long-standing relationship between the University and the Douglass Center (discussed in more detail in chapter 4) the University was of prime importance as a reference point for the center's clinical staff, especially the psychiatrists. Their relationship to the University was, however, ambivalent. The role of the Douglass Center as a training hospital, the fact that almost all its psychiatric staff were trained at the University, and the resources provided by the University were considered positive influences on the center. In addition, the University was related to the APU through the patients it sent to or received from it; sometimes the University's "psych wards" could be persuaded to take an "interesting" patient, and the University sent to the Douglass Center patients whose insurance had run out or whose unmanageability threatened their less restrictive operation.

For the APU staff, however, the University was also what might be called a source of contempt (Harre 1980). The University was a most desirable potential source of recognition from colleagues, yet the work carried out on the APU did not qualify for it. The patients were too "difficult" to be "rewarding" by University standards: one University psychiatrist, after a brief stint as a consultant, said that the Douglass Center patients were the "most awful" patients she had ever seen. Perhaps more importantly, the kind of work respected by many at the University—long-term, psychoanalytically oriented psychotherapy—was an impossibility on the unit.[16] Thus from the point of view of the psychiatrists who worked at the center, but were affiliated with the University, their colleagues seemed to regard them as doing the "dirty work" of psychiatry, work freely acknowledged on all sides to be difficult and undesirable. Only a few "mavericks" like Caldwell insisted that it was *their* work, more attractive to them than doing long-term psychotherapy with middle-class patients.

For the APU staff, the disappearance of Nolan was symbolic of their unit's position as an outpost; it represented one way in which the work could be satisfying. Certainly no one outside the unit seemed to them to appreciate the work involved in attaining such an ambiguous result. As Robert Naumann complained:

This job is very frustrating, especially the lack of positive feedback. Very few patients ever call you up and say, "I'm doing great." Maybe two out of a hundred if you're lucky. Instead, 35 percent come right back in the door again.

However, this lack of feedback and respect could be made into a perverse asset, with the staff taking an unorthodox pride in the unit's place in the scheme of things. This was the case with Nolan, who provided an opportunity to highlight the unit's situation. Ben and Sam often seized on minor events to make the point that while the unit's function was both necessary and unpleasant, "the enjoyment of unpleasant places" was always a possibility.

There was a sewage crisis on the unit over the weekend. On Monday morning Bea Radnor, the inpatient director, came down to ask about the drain, interrupting a staffing meeting. She rarely came to the unit and was greeted by much laughter from the staff (leaving her slightly nonplussed). After she left Sam said, "It' poetic justice; it makes clear to the external world our position. As long as we work OK, she can pretend we're not here, but when we get stopped up, the whole place stinks!"

Patients had to flow through the funnel, the drain, of the APU or the whole system would get clogged up. But since this function was invisible unless it failed, the unit had the positive attention of neither "regular" psychiatry nor the patients. The staff had no choice but to create themselves as their own audience.

The ambiguous relationship between the unit and the outside world suggests that many of the things that were described, especially in writing or when speaking formally, as nouns—aftercare, treatment options, disposition—were in fact verbs. The staff were actors enmeshed in a world of gestures; turfing, getting rid of, carrying jello, working out the puzzle pieces. Their gestures formed the connections in a complex field of strategic possibilities. Ben explained, for instance, that he saw Emergency Services as "a machine needing periodic adjusting; you do things, but you don't know if they'll work out. Understanding (e.g., of patients) turned out not to be it." The connections among gestures were ephemeral—they were between *this* social worker and *this* patient and *this* boarding home at this moment, and the arrangement could, and often did, fall apart and have to be reconstituted in a different form on a different day. This was why aftercare was neglected by the APU staff. The appointment written in a patients's chart did not show how tenuous and partial the arrangements were that got the patient out of the unit. The staff, however, generally knew that it did not reflect the patient's real relationship to the "system" in which he was (sometimes temporarily) embedded.

The staff's creation of themselves as their own audience and their immersion in the gestures required by the unit's orientation to direct action came together in the strategies they used to get patients out. It is to these I now turn.

THREE

The Game of Hot Shit

I

This is a shifty game: you have to seize opportunity as it arises.
—SAM WISHINSKI

The good thing about emergency problems is that they end. If they don't end, they can be defined as chronic and sent on to someone else.
—BEN CALDWELL

Shortly after I came to the unit, Sam saw a play about Admiral Scott's ill-fated expedition to the South Pole. Scott and all of his men died on the way back from the pole, having been beaten to it by a few days by the Norwegian explorer Amundsen. In the play *Terra Nova* (Tally 1981), Amundsen is a pragmatic man who taunts Scott with his unwillingness to bend to the practical exigencies of his situation. Scott, an Englishman, maintains to the end the strictest rules of gentlemanly decency. He refuses to use his dogs for food or to leave injured men behind. His actions have as their reference point the world he comes from, not the world he is in. There is, however, one moment when he looks out on the frozen wastes stretching away from his tent and says suddenly, as though seeing it for the first time, "Good God, this is an *awful* place!"

Sam felt this scene provided a useful image for understanding work on the APU. The unit was an "awful place" where the rules provided by the outside world were brought into question. The staff had to be like Amundsen, willing to pay attention to context even when it contradicted their expectations. Sam remembered a story he heard in college:

A man saw a sign in a shop window that said "We press pants." The next day he took in a pair of pants to be pressed. "Oh no," said the shopkeeper, "We don't press pants, we make signs."

In context, the sign made sense, but the context had to be known. Like the sign shop, the unit had to be entered, questions had to be asked, before the nature of its work could become evident.

Many staff members acknowledged that the unit could foster feelings of what Robert Naumann called "hopelessness and helplessness":

> There's a whole complex of political realities, things you can't accomplish because they're out of your control. There are real limitations and these shape you. Take somebody just out of the residency program, suddenly they're in a unit that's by definition short-term; the patients are poor, not motivated to change, and don't have the support systems or values you're used to . . . you wind up feeling totally powerless.

Ben, in a talk on emergency psychiatry to a group of residents, explained more formally:

> These jobs are closely related to our rescue fantasies, wanting to help people. As children we see ourselves as autonomous; later we realize we have to work in concert with other people. Things intrude on this fantasy—like impossible patients—and intrude on our capacity to do the work.

Ben taught residents and medical students that the "fantasy" had to be seen for what it was, an unrealistic image of solitary heroics, and the "intrusions" recast as a source (however difficult and unlikely) of satisfaction. The staff had to move from the position of Scott to the position of Amundsen; they had to learn to "eat their dogs."[1]

The comments of students showed that the unit challenged their initial ideas about rescuing patients. One student made this comment when he had been on the unit only a few days.

> There's nobody here that's relatable to—they're either so acute or so poor. And the patient I'm taking care of now has a lot to do with my [change of] attitude. She's eighteen and came from New York with drinking problems. I was excited about being able to help her. Later she got depressed and I felt really sad . . . But I kept talking to her. And she kept withholding information and was very uncooperative. So my attitude about her changed and I decided I didn't really care that much about her. I still have the idea they should do therapy [here] but it is a short-term unit. I think the staff are doing everything they can and they know what they're doing. I think it could be better but I don't know how it could be.

Frustrated by his patient's refusal to respond to his help, he decides that he doesn't "care for her" after all. Although he has a vague feeling that "the staff know what they're doing," that somehow they have become comfortable, he can't see *what* they have learned how to do. He still thinks they press pants. But within a couple of weeks this ambivalence gave way to a wholehearted enthusiasm for the goals of the unit.

> *I feel like I've really been integrated into the unit . . . We [have] this patient from Cleveland. [We should] interview him and find out if he understands the court (which he does)—he's insane but competent—watch him for a few days and send him back to jail; he'll get off. They'll send him home; he's got money from someplace, doesn't have a drug problem, and he has his own mission in life because he thinks he's the son of God.*

The emphasis has changed. The student is now interested in the efficiency with which the patient's situation can be handled. No longer concerned with his own feelings of "care" which proved fragile in the face of patients' behavior, he is optimistic about the patients' ability to survive and pragmatic about the role of the unit in the patient's life.

Other students expressed similar transformations in their perspective. A resident said:

> *I was scared at first. This is so different from the type of psychiatry I'm used to. You don't really talk to anyone [the patients]; you just cut through all the bullshit. One reason I like it here is that I never thought I did as much good [where I worked before]. Here I can see the utility of what I do.*

A medical student said after a few weeks on the APU:

> *Sam's task is not to be a magical, accessible therapist. He showed me that you can do more by not throwing patients in a vat of goodness and trying to straighten out everything for them, which was what I thought mental hospitals were all about . . . Getting rid of them is the point: What are you going to do with them?*

These students had to find ways of feeling capable and competent that did not depend on whether the patient shared their goals, got better, came back, or did not come back, or appreciated them. In Ben's talk to the residents he listed "feeling competent" as a primary goal for practitioners, one that he believed could be met if expectations were changed and the realities of the work faced squarely. But in order to feel competent the staff had to enter the "discourse on competence" (Good 1985:247) that was specific to the unit.[2] Rom Harre uses the term "hazard" to refer to social settings that test or challenge those who pass through them (1980:22–26). The APU was a "hazard" for its staff, challenging them to develop a local perspective on competence that would make their work possible, bearable, and, perhaps, enjoyable.

In order to develop this perspective the staff had to change their expectations of themselves and their patients. They talked of having learned what they could, and could not, accomplish. Barbara explained that:

> We are doing just what you'd expect [under the circumstances]. When the patient comes in you make a quick decision and make your plans. We don't get into their intrapsychic life; our goal is to reduce their anxiety.

Ronnie Lenahan said:

> I don't get discouraged. I accept that some patients will never get better and some will come back. I accept our limitations . . . no great expectations.

Ben explained that "it is a mistake to try to be capable," that is, to provide the kind of therapy and extended intervention that might be available in a different kind of place. Competence had to come from other sources.

A primary source was efficiency. The unit channeled the energy of the staff into an emphasis on speed and an awareness of their use of time and resources. Sam explained that:

> On the APU, quick treatment is part of the job. We don't pretend to our-selves or the patient that we are providing complete treatment; I say to patients, "You're not getting treated here." One patient said to me "You're here to expedite, not to alleviate." I said, "You're 100 percent right!"

The time of the staff was disciplined, not only by the internal structure of the unit, but also by the pressure of patients and the potential for getting "clogged." Those staff members who had been on the unit for a long time drew a sharp contrast between its proper, efficient use and its misuse as a "hideout" for patients who could manage outside. For instance, Sally said that she felt the unit should be a quick "in and out place" to stabilize patients, not offering them help with "secondary problems." Talking to me just before a weekend, she complained: "The whole hospital is full; now what will I do over the weekend? The APU is misused when it is treated as a haven; we should give [patients] meds and let them sit out in the lobby for an hour or so and send them home if they get better, not just let them in. That's what I'll have to do anyway over the weekend." In Sally's experience, to linger over any one patient simply deprived others.

The staff presented their efficiency as a contrast to other facilities (remember, for example, their contempt for the "dilly-dallying" of their New York counterparts when they wanted to get rid of Nolan). They stressed that they provided a peculiar but often appropriate kind of treatment, what Sam called a "harsh and undeceptive offering" that did not "infantalize" the patients. Sam compared it with a picture in his house of a rather angular and unyielding mother holding a child. "We should also be firm and ill-fitting," he said. "We treat the patients in a very tough way."

Although the APU staff emphasized their uniqueness, we can see that the unit's operation had much in common with other institutional forms that fill a space with a movement that produces a product. Factories, schools, and other institutions also have their roots in the efficient management of time. Work discipline in our society is intimately connected with a perception of time as a substance that can be manipulated in the service of production (Thompson 1967; Harvey 1985). In their management of the patients the staff rarely lost sight of the interplay between available beds and available time as the measure of their success. Walter Boyd compared the unit to television programs where a group of colleagues struggles with a difficult situation in a way that gets things done:

> This place is like M*A*S*H or Barney Miller. Just a conglomeration of people coming together who for some reason are efficient. It's too deep to make sense of "by the book."

"The book"—the official rules under which the unit operated—did not reveal the dynamic at the heart of the work, the satisfaction to be found in moving patients efficiently. As in the comedy shows, the unit's humor rested in part on the contrast between this instrumental and objective approach to the task and the contrary, pathetic, or resistant human "material" on which it was carried out.

Ben and Sam spoke of "relabeling patients from 'horrible' to 'unusual opportunity'" in order to persuade others to take them. They talked of "redefining" and "reframing" patients' situations to make them more amenable to change.[3] This notion of reframing can be extended to the unit's approach to competence and capability. The permanent staff engaged in a reframing of competence that emphasized the necessity to "act upon the actions of others" (Foucault 1983:223) primarily through the avenue of disposition. Action on the patients was seen in terms of its effect on the efficiency with which they could be moved through the unit. The staff did not expect their reward to come directly from the patients; instead they found it in interaction with other staff members who were engaged in the same task.

David Harvey speaks of the ways in which "urbanized human nature . . . is endowed with a very specific sense of space, time and money."

Taking shape in a partitioned, impersonal space and a disciplined, segmented time, this sensibility involves an uneasy reconciliation of the abstract (for example, money) and the concrete (daily life shaped by the use of money). Harvey suggests that a living out of this relationship of "concrete abstraction" occurs in the "hidden interiors" of urban life (1985:24). Using "sophisticated strategies . . . to win back from one corner of urban life what may be lost in another," people "find solace and hope in the intricacy of the game" (1985:35).

The APU staff used strategy to treat patients quickly and get them out efficiently, thus mastering the concrete abstraction of the unit's operation. The mastery of strategy enabled them to negotiate the unit's hazard as a workplace—the danger of falling into inefficiency and encountering the "pressure" of emergencies that built up, predictably but erratically, outside. This strategy in the service of disposition was part of a larger strategy that reframed competence, turning the work from a source of despair into the solace of mastering and sharing the task of disposition. The staff emphasized their difference from the rest of psychiatry partly to situate this reframing firmly in the here and now of the unit; as Ben said, "It's the attitude that we're unique that counts. Who cares whether we really are or not?"

The resolution achieved in efficiency was always partial. Patients resisted it; sometimes the administration undermined it. The staff found other ways to feel competent, as we see in the case study at the end of this chapter. But first we need to look at the way everyday practice on the unit took shape around the effort to produce empty beds.

II

I like working here, I like the pace and the rapid turnover. I like not having to work with patients for months.

—RONNIE LENAHAN

The house staff seemed to be constantly preoccupied with ways to get rid of patients.

—TERRY MIZRAHI (1986:85)

The staff of the APU congratulated themselves on keeping beds empty. For instance, Sam often announced a "score." He would say, "We're down to five, we're in good shape" or "We've got some leeway (before a weekend); we're not constipated." The staff were often reminded that their role in maintaining open beds was important to the hospital. About to go over several newly arranged dispositions, Sam would say cheerfully, "Here's how we will save the hospital!"

Much of the planning and negotiation that led to these successes took place at the meeting called "staffing" where, twice a week, ten to fifteen staff members gathered to discuss the patients. Staffing channeled the energy of the APU staff toward their common goal and provided an arena for showing off their skill. As Sam put it: "Staffing is solace." The meeting provided comfort through an exploration of the fields of action represented by the patients, who were both its object and its units of communication.

The staffing meeting was structured to take up the case of each patient in turn. The meeting was led by Sam, who guided the discussion, proposed solutions, and wrote plans for the patient in a small notebook. In these discussions the staff developed their knowledge about the patient, sharing what they knew and simultaneously probing into the patient's situation, and exploring possible placements. Knowledge of the patient's situation, condition, and response to the unit provided the staff with the material basis for making plans, and plans depended on the staff's knowledge and skill in finding a likely "match" between the patient and the outside world. Staffing discussions revolved around the contingent and diffuse nature of both knowledge and planning; each patient was a puzzle to be fitted into a larger puzzle, and the task was to find the point at which these two "puzzle pieces" (to use Robert Naumann's term) articulated.

This task was a matter of contextualization and depended on the specific details of each case. Often the discussion of a patient ended with a series of "if . . . then" statements by Sam that summed up all the possibilities and strategies that had been discussed: "OK, if his charges are dropped, then . . . and if that doesn't work, then . . ." Sam guided the staff to look for the links between their limited knowledge of the patient and the limited possibilities for an immediate solution. Over the period of minutes, days, or weeks that a patient came up in staffing, he worked through the steps ("Consider keeping him until Monday," "Let's get his charges dropped," "Pull the old chart") that would lead to a realistic disposition. What was reasonable depended on what the staff could find out about the patient and on what they knew of the available places and their power to gain entry to them.

The discussions that took place in staffing were often fragmentary and lacking in resolution. They did not provide coherent narratives about patients, nor did they point to consistencies in the way the staff handled specific problems. In fact, the staff took up bits and pieces of patients' histories and situations in such a way that a decision about one patient might contradict that for another. The guiding principle was the uncovering of that aspect of the patient essential to the next step in moving toward a disposition.

The staff did not always discharge a patient at the earliest opportunity. Their decision depended on whether other beds were available on the unit and on whether the patient appeared likely to benefit from a few additional days of hospitalization. For instance, a patient who had not responded to medication within the first two or three days on the unit might receive a change of medication and be retained for several additional days to see whether the change had an effect. The staff believed that such a patient, once sent to a longer-term unit, would get "stuck" there regardless of need; when they had room, they preferred to wait and see whether the patient could be discharged altogether.

Staffing was structured around the presentation of each patient, in turn, as a "case." If the patient was new, Sam read directly from the admitting note in the chart; if the patient was already on the unit his progress was reported, usually by the student assigned to him.[4] These presentations combined the formal language of psychiatry with more casual comments. For example:

■   The patient is a 34-year-old black male, carrying a diagnosis of paranoid schizophrenia, who was brought in by his brother for evaluation because of his bizarre behavior . . . he talks in riddles, says he's a "Sheep led astray in a sea of glass" [Sam says, *sotto voce*, "Oh boy!"].

The chart provided a starting point for exploring the patient's mental state, which was expressed in terms of diagnosis (organic brain syndrome, paranoid schizophrenia) and behavior (pressured speech, poor hygiene). Usually the chart also provided some information on the patient's relationship to other agencies and to family supports:

■   [The patient] originally presented at screening . . . they sent him to [another local hospital] for admission but after five or six days [that hospital] sent him back here.

The simplest resolution of a screening presentation was a question [usually from Sam] pointing to a single move leading directly to discharge.

RESIDENT: This patient, who was brought in by police, was raking a relative's yard and drank a fifth of gin while he was doing it. He doesn't remember what happened after that and we don't know either.

SAM: He's out of withdrawal danger. Is he competent now?

RESIDENT: He seems pretty competent. Medication seems to help a little.

SAM [writing in his book]: Evaluate competency and send him back [to jail] this afternoon.

Usually more extensive discussion was required to make the situation clear. This did not follow a predictable format, but involved a loose, sometimes digressive, consideration of various facets of the case.

DUANE: I wonder if we're messing the patient up with drugs. He had akathesia; he's stiff [these are side effects of neuroleptics]. Maybe his meds are causing his symptoms. If he's got private insurance we're gonna get rid of him. I met his mother yesterday; there's no precipitating factor that she knows of.

SAM: I think the mother is a precipitating factor: her indecision.

DUANE: Her whole behavior is strange.

Sam talks about the patient's anxiety about separation in relation to the mother's behavior.

DUANE: His touching and grabbing people fits with what you describe.

ANOTHER RESIDENT [to Sam]: What do you mean by symbiotic psychosis?

SAM: It's a term used by Mahler and described very well in *The Psychological Birth of the Human Infant* (1975). [He gives an example of a child who couldn't deal with separation and named her doll "urgy mergy."] . . . Here, you could make a case that the mother is behaving unreasonably and making him worse. If he's got insurance, work toward private hospitalization. With her, work with her denial [that there is a problem]; she may be unresponsive to any rational approach. If he doesn't have insurance he should go upstairs.

DUANE: Seclusion makes him worse.

SAM: That's a good observation. Seclusion is bad for separation problems.

DUANE: But he's hard on the staff. But I'm gonna write not to seclude him and to reduce his meds.

LILLIAN: What should we do when he kicks the doors, restraint or what? [spoken from an awareness that, in fact, the use of restraint was not permitted on the unit]

SAM: He may require one to one nursing at times.

WALTER: If he's going up and touching people, especially paranoid patients, he's liable to get popped!

SAM: You're bringing up the other side. But we can make an effort to try other things before we put him in seclusion where he might freak out.

In this discussion it is as though the group is shining a rapidly moving light over all the different aspects of the case; sometimes the light falls on an area of coherence, where there is a match between the patient's behavior and psychoanalytic theory, or between the patient's problems and an overdose of medication. Some of these areas suggest possibilities for action. The residents and Sam were interested in the psychological dynamics of the case. But they did not allow theoretical speculation to take them very far from the practical realities—the patient's medication, potential for disrupting the ward, and options for discharge. Separation problems were interesting, but separation from the unit was paramount.

The separation of the patient from the unit depended in part on two characteristics of the patient himself: reaction to medication and motivation. In most cases the staff saw these as areas where they could have an immediate effect on the patient's behavior. Medication and motivation were sometimes related, as when a patient returned to the hospital after stopping medication on his own; when motivation failed, medication remained as the most direct route, via the patient's body, to a change of mind. This route was attractive to the staff because of its materiality and potential for fast results, but it was not without pitfalls.

SAM [of an older patient admitted by one of the residents from a ward upstairs]: How is her depression?

RESIDENT: Yesterday she was very happily depressed. I wanted to see if the stress of the APU would help get her out of the hospital. But she's been very quiet, so I thought I'd bump her upstairs for a short visit and up her meds to the max.

SAM: Have you seen the article in the *New England Journal* about psychotropic drugs for the elderly? Sometimes they get more agitated [that is, worse] the higher the dose.

Sometimes, in other words, reducing the medication could have as much effect as increasing it. The following discussion is about a patient who had just been transferred from another hospital where he had become assaultive.

DUANE: He woke up after I took him off Thorazine [chlorpromazine, an antipsychotic] . . . like a new man. He had been on a lot of Thorazine, really doped up, a zombie.

SAM: That was revenge [from the hospital that had transferred him]. He lit a fire in the day room and assaulted their staff.

DUANE: I took him off Thorazine. [Mischievously] I gave him some matches and put him on Prolixin.

SAM: By the way, that's what Minuchin [a well-known family therapist] does with child fire-setters.

ANOTHER RESIDENT: Send 'em to State Hospital?

SAM: He gives them matches and instructions on how to use.

MEDICAL STUDENT: We don't have to worry about fires here; there's nothing to burn.

SAM: This is a terrific workup [report] from [the other hospital]. It's as if they are saying to us: look at our workup, why don't you do as well?

DUANE: They really snowed the patient [gave a high dose of drugs]. That must be a terrible feeling.

From the staff perspective, the other hospital looked good on paper, but its staff had not had the facilities ("nothing to burn") or the sense of humor to handle the patient. In this discussion we can see one of Sam's strategies for reframing an event; by whimsically suggesting an absurd or extreme possibility (give the patient matches) and referring it to an outside authority, he opens up the situation to humorous or unconventional interpretations.

With a different patient, just the opposite effect might be desired from medication.

WALTER: The patient says that Haldol makes him feel like a zombie.

DUANE: That's the ticket; that's where we want him.

In many cases the question of where to place a patient depended on what the patient could or would do for herself. For example, was a patient likely to attend day treatment if she was sent home, or could she follow the regulations in a boarding house? The staff used staffing to volunteer their experiences with and opinions about a patient, to offer speculations about motivation, and to calibrate or modify their efforts.

They did "detective work" in an attempt to see into the truth about the patient.

■   This 20-year-old patient sleeps in shelters, has a drinking problem and was kicked out by his parents who say he's strange. He only needs a few days for evaluation of (the effect of) neuroleptics.,

SAM: Is he a day treatment candidate?

RESIDENT: Maybe. He seems fairly unmotivated.

■   The patient is an alcoholic with multiple hospitalizations who came in with suicidal ideation. He has stated that he does not intend to stop drinking or go to AA.

LILLIAN: So he did come in for a vacation.

RESIDENT: Yeah, that's why I'm discharging him . . . I'm a little cynical about this guy.

When the staff felt that the patient was capable of cooperating with a plan, they did not shrink from direct confrontation on issues of responsibility.

SAM: The question [about this patient] was disposition, wasn't it?

SOCIAL WORKER: He's gonna be a disposition problem wherever he goes because of his noncompliance. The group home fell through. We're considering another place.

LILLIAN: We want to talk to him first about his seriousness [about going to a home]. Rules and regulations are important in a boarding home. We just want to have a heart to heart talk with him. He will have to negotiate what happens.

DUANE: I don't think he was that bad when he came in, more lonely than anything else. His aunt is just sort of throwing her hands up and dumping him here. This boarding home is his last chance.

LILLIAN: That's the heart to heart we're gonna have.

Lillian, who was aware that a patient's behavior might result in the burning of his last bridge, often warned less experienced staff away from believing everything they heard from patients.

RESIDENT: When I tried to talk to [the patient] about alternatives he talked about needing structure, so I thought of sending him upstairs [to one of the longer-term wards].

LILLIAN: Does he want a structured program because he has a need, or because he's lazy? We [social workers] spoke to him a couple of times and we had the impression he wanted everything on a silver platter . . . I don't know if I want to pursue a dependent type of situation. I told him: Do you think I'm going to cure you? I'm not that type of social worker!

"That type of social worker" does "everything" for the patient, and patients accustomed to such attention were, in Lillian's view, sometimes disappointed not to find themselves in a "dependent-type situation."

The staff often had to explore many sources of information; sometimes the patient was one of the least important. In this case, the patient's family, her behavior, and her previous [Douglass Center] chart are all potential sources.

LILLIAN: Let's start with Johnson.

MEDICAL STUDENT: She was doing much better. She should probably leave soon.

DUANE [coming in]: You talking about Johnson?

LILLIAN: I'll call her home today, see where she can stay.

DUANE: She's better? We'll keep her down here [because she can leave soon].

SOCIAL WORK STUDENT: She's hiding her food, says she's not Johnson, her name is a secret.

DUANE: She doesn't sound better to me.

LILLIAN: We need her old chart [to get a better sense of whether she will improve quickly].

DUANE: Well, you don't have to send her upstairs today if you think she's getting better. See how she does.

In this conversation, the staff see their job as an attempt to have an immediate impact on this patient. If she improved quickly, she "belonged" on the unit because she could leave quickly; if she appeared to be a long-term case, she needed to be sent elsewhere.

Changing the medication and exploring the motivation of a patient were relatively unambiguous approaches; in many cases neither could be counted on to get a patient out. The staff sometimes indicated that what was required was not so much a change in the patient as a change in the definition of the problem. For example, Sam is talking about an old woman who was disturbing the other patients.

> *We can send her back to State Hospital. The troublesome symptom is that she screams all night. If we redefine the problem as disturbing the ward, then we can aim not to cure her but to remove the symptom with Restoril.*

However, a patient could seem better than the staff knew he really was.

STUDENT [referring to a patient]: I don't know what to do with him.

SAM: He doesn't look too bad, which is the problem. He doesn't look certifiable even though he does threaten people. Maybe he should go to jail.

Even the effects of medication could, in some circumstances, be regarded as a matter of appearance. In general, the staff looked to the calming effects of medication as positive; the effectiveness of medication was taken for granted and rarely discussed. Sometimes, however, medications were used in a paradoxical way; it was occasionally considered to the advantage of the patient and the unit not to change a patient's behavior immediately. This occurred when a patient needed to be free of medication in order to make a diagnosis. Sometimes the patient's continuing symptoms were needed to ensure retention through the legal system.

RESIDENT: I'm going to put off adjusting her neuroleptics until after the hearing. I've had problems with giving too much [thus sedating the patient] and having the patient released.

RESIDENT: I just kept her crazy . . . so she'll be sent to State Hospital today.

Because hearings only occurred once a week, a patient who could maintain a noncrazy appearance for a few minutes on that one day might be able to slip through the legal net and get released despite her psychosis.

We can see in these examples that the question of disposition was woven into discussion of patients from the beginning. It did not form a separate issue to be decided after other things were in place. Disposition required of staff that they change whatever could be quickly changed about a patient, that they accept and act quickly when patients did not improve, that they know what was available, and that they know how to make the match work. This demanded cunning on their part and, sometimes, help from the patient.

Often Sam pointed out to the residents and students what they should look for in terms of disposition. For example, he used the phrase "Aha, family!" whenever family members were mentioned and encouraged the staff to find out whether the family could be persuaded to take the patient or if the patient would go to the family.

SAM: Let's tell [this patient] that Lillian and [the social work student] are going to go out and try to find her family and find out why her sister threw her out.

The legal system also provided openings and possibilities that might not be immediately evident to students. Sometimes a patient could be sent back to stand trial; once evaluated and declared competent a patient was no longer the responsibility of the unit. But of course a clearly deranged or incompetent patient would just bounce back within a few hours, days, or months. For such patients, the legal charges themselves might exert a leverage unrelated to their content, or function to influence other parts of the system.

SAM [to student]: If the patient is willing to stay, drop charges, if not, don't drop charges. If she won't sign a voluntary and is not certifiable, we maintain charges in order to keep her.

In other words, this was a patient who seemed to need hospitalization (and could perhaps be transferred upstairs) but might not be willing to stay voluntarily. The criminal charges served as a useful, if crude and temporary, restraint. The following example is more complex. This patient was brought from jail; he was clearly incompetent but his identity was unknown.

SAM: Let's not drop charges quite yet because with his charges we may be able to get his fingerprints [and thus his identity]. The police are more likely to do that [for us] if he has charges.

The staff called the kind of maneuver evidenced in this last example "active ignorance" or "creative naivete." In some cases it was not in their interest to use all that they knew.

LILLIAN: This issue [the discharge of a patient who had been at the state hospital] is political. We will never get patients [back] into State Hospital if we let them go, even though he *could* make it on the outside.

STUDENT: Well, we don't *have* to treat elevated affect! [In other words, "We can just keep him crazy."]

The staff also had occasion to conceal or omit information that might make a patient unacceptable to a particular placement.

SAM: None of us expect him to be compliant with day treatment.

LILLIAN: They don't like people who don't show up.

SAM: I think we should be creatively naive about him; assume he'll be OK and be surprised when he shows up here again [after failing at day treatment].

Difficult and hard to place patients stretched the ability of the staff, requiring intricate strategies involving both the expectations of others at the Douglass Center and the demands of other agencies. Here is a particularly subtle example:

■ The patient is an old woman with senile dementia. The chronic care facility connected with the state hospital had agreed to take her "when she is not agitated," putting the unit in a bind since her agitation was the reason they wanted to transfer her in the first place. In the meantime the inpatient director, Bea Radnor, had told the social worker to "work with the family." This conventional piece of advice, according to Sam, "betrays a misunderstanding of the function of this unit and overlooks the fact that we are full and the needs of the hospital." At this point Sam outlined a strategy: "Here's the way we'll turn it around. Pull the chart and see what medication worked the last time. We will then step on that. Contact the chronic care unit [independently] before Dr. Y [director of the state hospital section responsible for admissions from the Douglass Center to the chronic unit] can reach them. Say you want to postpone the admission for a few days because she needs a sonogram and we will do it and save them the trouble [thus the issue of "agitation" is neatly bypassed while gaining a couple of days to sedate the patient]. *Then* we can contact Dr. Y and say that we are happy to hear that he will accept her now that the chronic care unit is willing."

In this strategy the staff played two parts of the state hospital against each other (the long-term ward itself and the inpatient director) while they bought time in which to change the patient's condition with medication.

When something like this worked the staff expressed a complex mixture of pride, relief, and guilt. A few days later, when this patient was successfully transferred, people discussed how hard it would be for the state hospital to find a further placement for her.

SAM: Well, it's their problem now.

LILLIAN: That makes me feel better! [To nurse] Write on her chart, scrawl something illegible.

Concealed behind the scrawl on the chart were the weaknesses of other facilities, the ignorance of outside agencies, and the guilt of patients' families. Anything that might open up a place was considered, and subterfuge was sometimes a necessary part of the game.

Here is one final example of strategizing, which shows how the process began as soon as a patient was admitted, and how quickly several solutions were explored. The patient was young, with a history of previous admissions, "cooperative but psychotic."

RONNIE: Is he the one that follows B [another patient] around, goes into his room, and sits and grins? [everyone laughs]

SAM [to student]: Why don't you find out his baseline, how far he is from his usual level of functioning.

WALTER: Not far.

RONNIE: His brother and sister visited on Friday.

SAM: Ah! Family! [to student] Try to contact the family and check the old chart to see what his meds were and compare with what we have him on now. Also ask him if he can sign a voluntary, maybe we can take him off certs . . . No, perhaps we should keep his certs in order to get him out more easily . . .

The APU staff had to accept that their work involved elements of uncertainty that planning could not overcome.[5] They did not know how a discharged patient would react, whether another facility, or his family, would accommodate him, or whether he and those around him would be safe. To some extent Sam, Lillian, Ronnie, and Walter demonstrated in staffing what they considered acceptable levels of risk. They showed residents and other newcomers the narrow limits within which they could control the behavior of future of patients, for, as Light has pointed out, in psychiatry residents "do not know the outcomes of decisions and actions by themselves or others" (1980:292). They helped those who were initially disconcerted by the unit to develop a local perspective that highlighted what could be done and muted what could not. And they sometimes pulled eager students back from an oversimplified adoption of the very perspective they were teaching—for example, Sam, in one particular case, in response to the staff's disgust with a cocaine-addicted patient, insisted that a student think about follow-up.

In the following discussion Walter and Sam directly address the most serious, and also rarest, risk they faced, that of injury or death in the hospital itself. This discussion shows that they perceive uncertainty to have two layers, the first being that of the uncertainty surrounding the patient's behavior itself and the second the effect of the patient's behavior in exposing them to scrutiny. A patient on a ward upstairs jumped from a fourth-story window and was seriously injured.

WALTER: I'm a little itchy; it seems like these incidents are getting closer. I'm being overly cautious with everyone who comes in [to be admitted], as though someone's looking over my shoulder. The situation this month has been really heavy; we've had some really crazy folks.

SAM: The shells keep hitting and getting closer, and we're very vulnerable because we handle so many people and send so many out. I don't want to become immobilized; part of what lets us work is this devil-may-care nonchalance. If we ever think about what we're doing we wouldn't be able to do it. . . . Fortunately no one could get hurt falling out of *our* windows.

As in the discussion about the fire-setting patient, the unit's physical set-up is an advantage; it is too close to the ground (and too hard to get out of) for a patient to get hurt. But, more importantly, the efficiency of the unit requires that the staff not think too hard (once they have minimized the risks); "paralysis" would make the work impossible. Sam's war metaphor resembles Ben's description of the "invasion" of the unit by "virulent bacteria"; these images of the unit as a target suggested a vulnerability that, Sam implies, was best kept in the background.

Uncertainty was more often phrased as an awareness of the limits inherent in the task of placement. Many patients posed insoluble dilemmas, Catch 22 situations that never felt complete.

SAM [of a patient who is asking to leave]: We're trying to solve something we can't here. He's a chronic patient. The reality is we don't feel he can take care of himself, and he does. Let's transfer him upstairs.

LILLIAN: If you can talk him into it, fine, but he wants to go back to work . . .

ROBERT NAUMANN [of a patient admitted on certification]: I don't think he's actually dangerous. All he's done is verbal overtures. Yes, he's hallucinating. But he can go and hallucinate out there.

■ A patient is refusing to eat and refusing medication:

SAM: Transfer him and get his charges dropped. Let them worry about him. Let's find out what area he's in.

■ A patient who has been arrested for attempted burglary [he broke into a building, then fell asleep] can only get his charges dropped if he is under continued treatment. In the meantime, he wants to go to New York with his father.

DUANE: He says he doesn't need inpatient care but he will go to outpatient. He is unreliable and we can't tell the D.A. that he will go. Also, there's the property damage; I can't see how you can ship him back to New York.

SAM: He needs to go to court with a plea of guilty by reason of insanity.

DUANE: No, he knew what he was doing. He got *caught* by reason of insanity.

SAM: I don't see a way out of this. If he is guilty by reason of insanity he'll be sent to a long-term hospital. If he goes back to jail he'll keep coming back over and over . . . Seriously, we have to question whether deinstitutionalization is an appropriate goal for such people. For now we have to be unidealistic about this guy . . . maybe lie to the D.A.

[Duane shakes his head.]

SAM: We have an honest man in our midst, which is going to cost the state an untold amount of money. Anything we do is going to be wrong. Well, let's just do one very simple thing for today, anything . . .

DUANE: But we have to meet the father.

SAM: That's just an educational experience for you.

There was no way out of these situations. Even when patients left the unit, the sense of resolution came only from having somehow moved them on. The staff rarely discovered what happened to them unless they come back.

In staffing the APU staff helped one another through the "hazard" that the unit represented. Dealing with each patient as an individual puzzle, they worked out the limits of what they could do, dealt with issues of treatment and management, and aided one another in finding cunning solutions to intractable problems. They treated the patient and the outside world as fields of knowledge and power, in which fragments of information could be matched and juggled in the service of strategy. They celebrated their skill at using everything at hand, including the contradictions and absurdities that inevitably emerged from this task. At the same time, patients and events challenged this sense of competence and required other readings of the unit's work.

III

TURF: get rid of . . .

—SAMUEL SHEM (1978:428)

One day in July the director of a local nursing home brought a patient into screening and left him there, leaving the building before the screening nurse realized what had happened.

The patient's name was Charles Judge. He was in his early fifties, but he looked at least sixty-five. An alcoholic all his life, he suffered from brain damage. Though he had a dignified appearance, he was unable to care for himself; he could not speak more than a few words, had fits of falling down and lying on the floor, and was sometimes incontinent. The nursing home had found him unmanageable despite its use of restraints to keep him from wandering around.

Judge stayed on the APU for more than five months. He was an anomaly and, for this reason, he came to represent to the staff many aspects of their situation. He was a patient they couldn't get rid of, thereby highlighting the nature of their strategies and the essence of their relation to the outside world. At the same time, they developed a relationship with him that became paradigmatic of their ability to resist, when they had to, the unit's definition as an emergency facility. Through their redefinition of Judge as a "child" and a "pet" they collaborated to create an alternative image of the unit.[6]

The APU had already had two experiences of having patients from the nursing home "dumped" on them. This time Ben wanted to prove once and for all that these were inappropriate "referrals." He wrote an eight-page evaluation documenting that Charles Judge was not a psychiatric patient and admitted him on "holding status," which meant that he had no chart but was to be "held." Usually, this category was only used for a few hours for patients about to be transferred to other facilities. Ben liked the fact that he had such an obvious and well-witnessed case and hoped to "nail" the nursing home director and the Department of Mental Health on it. Talking later about his reaction to Charles Judge, Ben said: "When he came in I had two separate and contradictory feelings. One was, he should be in a state hospital, preferably in the old days when they had farms. And the other was, too bad, that's not what I'm the agent for, I'm the agent for a different set of values." One of these values was the protection of his unit from an influx of "inappropriate" admissions. Said Ben: "I wanted Sam *not* to solve [Judge's case] or we would have more of these problems to solve."

Judge was an inappropriate admission because he didn't have what staff considered a psychiatric disorder. They felt that he had a medical illness, dementia secondary to alcoholism. This illness was incurable and rendered him completely helpless. In addition, of course, he was without the resources to pay for his own care. Sam said:

> When Judge came in he was defined as the offal—the piece of shit in the game of hot potato, or hot shit, among parts of the system. Whoever got stuck with him would be the person who takes care of the shit. What do you call those people in Japan? The eta. Are psychiatrists the eta? Or nursing homes? The chronic wards? The community?

The initial reaction of the staff to Charles's admission was resentment.

SAM: I tried to avoid him. I said to the resident, this case has too many administrative complexities. I let him manage it.

WALTER [who was assigned to take care of Judge on a daily basis]: Initially when he came in he was a headache. He was a square peg trying to fit into a round hole. Not much we could do for him, and not much he could do for himself, either.

For the first month or more, Judge was an invisible patient. He had no official chart (though the staff kept an unofficial one), and he was not even discussed in staffing. When he was finally mentioned, it was with a certain defiance.

SAM: On Judge, there's nothing new. We're still awaiting word from the Department of Mental Health [on how to resolve the dispute with the nursing home]. Well, we won't do a thing, just see how long we can keep him here before anyone *does* anything.

At this point, Charles Judge represented for the staff their position as the drain and unconscious of psychiatry. No one seemed to see that they had taken him in, nor could they get the attention of those with the power to resolve the situation.

During the fall, the APU staff tried to exercise their competence at what they did best. They tried every possible option for disposition. Charles could not be accepted by home-care programs because he needed too much care, even if his niece, who lived in the city, had been willing to have him. For a while it looked as though a diagnosis of mental retardation might get him into a home for the retarded.

LILLIAN: I'm going to try to get through to the Mental Retardation program; I'll call Dr. D. first to find out how to present it to them.

SAM [hopefully]: We could have [the psychologist] test him. I'm sure he'd score retarded now.

But this fell through. The program only accepted retarded people who had been wrongly diagnosed as mentally ill, not those with organic brain damage. Sam joked in staffing, "We could interview his niece, she's not too swift. Maybe we could establish some genetic [tendency]." But, as Walter remarked later, "[There was] a painful side [to Judge's case]. We made light of it, but we were very aggressive in trying to get him out. It was a blow to my ego dealing with him because we're used to getting people out at a rapid pace."

In the meantime, Charles Judge was becoming a fixture on the unit; people were getting used to him.

SAM [in staffing]: I think everyone's getting comfortable with him here. I think if he gets very ill, Ben and Giuliani will get scared he'll die here and do something about him.

WALTER: He sleeps late, he's been hoarding stuff under his bed, ice cream, soda. So we have to watch it. But he's been up.

As this conversation indicates, there was concern, for a while, about his health, as he seemed to be going into a decline.

WALTER: I took him to the ER (Emergency Room) Friday. They said he was dehydrated. His teeth are bad.

SAM: Maybe we should try a softer diet, milkshakes.

LILLIAN: That [his teeth] is not making him feel good.

SAM: There used to be a time when they pulled the teeth of chronic inmates.

WALTER: He was angry at me for taking him to the ER. [Walter imitates Judge trying to say "You bastard."]

SAM: Does he look depressed?

WALTER: He's down, stays in his room a lot.

By calling up the image of the old hospital/prison and its toothless inmates, Sam throws into relief the care the staff are giving Mr. Judge. They want him to be "up," walking around in the safety of APU environment, in contrast to the nursing home where he was kept in restraints.

As this last conversation suggests, Walter, who was most involved in Judge's daily care, had by this time become the interpreter of his moods.

The staff had ceased to remain aloof from their patient's humanity. Sam said: "Eventually I felt uncomfortable about this man lying on the floor. It was hard to pretend he wasn't there. One of the great moments was when we finally got his niece in with her baby and Judge's eyes lit up and he talked to the baby—'dadada'!" Judge was like a child.

The staff began to talk as though they had a special understanding of Judge's needs.

WALTER: We're checking out the VA. They said to document that he's not a behavior problem. He has "seizures" and slides to the floor, but if he's ignored he goes to his room.

RONNIE: We walk right over him!

WALTER: If you say, "Want a drink?" he'll get up. Going to an old folks home is not good for him, no one would joke around with him.

SAM: So you're recommending nursery school?

RONNIE: Remember the baby? They got along perfectly—"dadada!"

Walter talked about the way his attitude toward Judge shifted as he accepted the hopelessness of the situation:

> *Things didn't lessen and there was no end in sight. [Judge] became a continual headache. Then I got empathetic, though still annoyed. I was beyond the point of being angry at being imposed on; it became a routine, knowing we didn't have any alternatives.*

At this point, the implications of Judge's name began to be felt. Sam said, "Then we lose, we've got him. But then he becomes a human being, we realize he's not a piece of shit. He's *The Judge.*

Judge's health improved, and staff were proud of their success. As Walter put it "We're doing good work; the Judge is getting better." When Thanksgiving came around Judge's family wanted him to come home for the day. But Ben and Sam decided against it. Ben was worried that Judge might overeat and get sick. And, on principle, he felt that "they can't just take him when they feel like it; we will not provide an interim rest home for the family." Here again Ben was interested in defining the limits of the unit's role. But there was also the sense in which Judge had become like a child to the staff; they defended him against the competing, but erratic, attentions of his family.

Increasingly, the Judge was accepted as he was. He was always the last to be brought up in staffing, a recurring addendum to the normal business of moving people along, often greeted with the (by now) timeworn joke: "Here come de Judge!" Staff still felt their failure to place him as a challenge to their competence, but they also found that treating the Judge as a guest had its own rewards. Enjoyment of his personality began to change into feelings of self-respect for the appreciation and care they were giving him. Sam recalled later: "Judge would play in the bathtub which endeared him to us. At first it was seen as a behavior problem because he didn't want to get out, but we redefined it that he enjoyed it and started putting him in there to play and sing." The staff were proud that Judge's "wandering," "fits," and babbling were not problematic for them.

By late November the Judge was a fixture on the unit. All attempts to place him had failed. Sometimes now he was referred to as a "pet."

■   [In the Day Room] Judge, who has been sitting at the table, suddenly starts to lean to one side with his eyes closed. Another patient tries to stop him. Trina, the direct care worker, says, "One thing about the Judge, he never falls." The other patient asks, "Is he sick?" "Yeah," says Trina, "we have real sick people in here. This is a mental hospital." She says to me, "The Judge, he's Sally's [the head nurse] pet, that's why he's still here."

At this point Giuliani became concerned about the use of "holding status" to keep a patient indefinitely. He consulted legal authorities at the state level, who said that this practice was probably illegal. To make the situation look better, Ben abolished "holding status," replacing it with a new category called "awaiting disposition." (On hearing about this the resident said to Sam, "Same rules apply?" "Of course," said Sam.) The only way out of holding the Judge seemed to be the one that was rejected at the beginning to make the point, that is, to give him a legal status and transfer him to a long-term unit.

A hearing was scheduled for the Judge. He was taken upstairs, looking neat and dignified. In the hearing room he sat straight and seemed to listen as Ben presented the problem, describing how he was admitted as a "guest" and could not be placed; Ben emphasized his complete inability to care for himself. The public defender asked Judge: "Do you want to stay here?" nodding as he said it, and Judge said "Yes," nodding back (he nodded "yes" to anything). Ben presented his doubts about voluntary admission since Judge would not understand what he was signing. But the hearing officer thought it was the only solution. He recommended that Judge be signed into the unit as a "voluntary" patient.

■   When they get back to the unit from the hearing Lillian asks Judge, "Do you want to stay?" Judge's head seems to clear and he says: "I want to get out of here." "Where would you go?" "I've got a place to go . . . I've got four . . ." says Judge, but then he falters. He can't remember the names of his children.

When this incident was described to Ben—it suggested that Judge did not want to stay—he said "I don't care, I'm keeping him." Judge's human needs had won out over the administrative agenda; it seemed pointless to make an issue of the involuntary quality of his "voluntary" admission.

Sam outlined the larger picture:

> *He became human to us. Clearly the Judge belongs on a decent chronic care unit. But the history of the mental health movement has distorted our faculties so we can't reach those elementary decisions. Instead, the medical establishment says he's psychiatric, psychiatry says it's medical . . . The Department of Mental Health says it doesn't matter what you say because we are implementing deinstitutionalization as a policy.*

Judge did "sign" a "voluntary" and, since there were no long-term beds available at the state hospital, he was transferred a few days later to a ward upstairs.

For Ben, whose mind was on administrative consequences, Judge represented the fact that, ultimately, anyone could be placed. For him, the unit's power rested in the confidence of the staff that all patients had a "niche."

> *I don't believe anything different about the Judge now . . . just another guy, no different from others who tramp through here, they all have a niche to which we can send them.*

But for most of the staff he became paradigmatic of their capacity to be flexible; they developed their own local, situated understanding of this patient for whom they had struggled so long to find a place. By the time the Judge left the unit he had become a source of self-congratulation for the staff and a category had been generated to describe him. He was no longer someone "awful" who "doesn't belong here" but a "pet," "someone we give good care to."

SAM: Gradually the fact that no other place can deal with him becomes the system's fault. We perceive the awfulness of the system instead of his awfulness. So he becomes a test case, a Judge.

A few months after Judge's departure Lillian reported with delight that he had finally been accepted into a long-term ward at the state hospital. In the meantime his history had become part of the unit's incorporation of new students. One day in staffing a patient was referred to as a "young Charles Judge." The new resident said, wistfully, "I wish I could meet the Judge."

Charles Judge was one point of articulation in a field of intersecting interests, strategies, and definitions. Each point in this field had its strength, its ability to exert force, and its weakness. The hospital could admit and yet not admit Judge; Ben could strategically refuse to solve the problem yet solve it after all (or was it a solution?); Sam could hold still, defiantly, to force action from above, yet he could not *not* act; the staff could strategize through diagnostic manipulations while pretending Judge did not exist. And it would demean the Judge not to accord him his mite of power as well, for he eluded restraints and, by sheer force of personality, found a temporary lodging.

The Judge also presented the staff with a space for commentary. They used irony, whimsy, and the outrageous expression of feeling to create him as a pet and a child, inverting conventional categories and making of him someone good to think with. As "hot shit," he represented their position in the mental health system; as "pet," their provision of a safe, if stark, haven, and as "child," their ability to nurture. As "the Judge," he was a silent witness both to the "awfulness" of "the system" itself and to the impossible task they were required to carry out. Thus the Judge became, through his anomalous and ambiguous position, a fruitful source of the imaginative construction of local understanding.

FOUR

History Modifies
Our Fantasies

I

*The illusory expectations that are associated with certain social deci-
sions . . . may keep their real future effect from view.*

—Albert Hirschman (1977:131)

Actual history modifies our fantasies.

—Ben Caldwell

In 1963, President Kennedy gave a Message to Congress in which he
proposed a radical reorientation of the nation's delivery of psychiatric
care:

> If we launch a broad new mental health program now, it will be possible
> within a decade or two to reduce the number of patients now under custodial
> care by 50 percent or more. Many more mentally ill can be helped to remain
> in their own homes without hardship to themselves or their families. Those
> who are hospitalized can be restored to useful life. (Levine 1981:52)

The Douglass Center is heir to this latest in a long series of attempts to
reform psychiatric treatment.[1] At the same time, it operates in an atmosphere of growing criticism of deinstitutionalization. This chapter is
about the history of the APU as it is told by the staff; their accounts are
expressive of the uncertain relationship between plans and results that
characterizes the history of psychiatry itself.

The asylum emerged in the early nineteenth century in conjunction
with attempts to reform the treatment of the insane (Foucault 1973,
Scull 1979).[2] The orderly architecture and systematic regimen called
moral treatment by early asylum doctors was believed to have a direct

effect on the disorderly minds of patients; the asylum was an embodiment of restraint (Foucault 1973, 1979, Rothman 1971). The evolution of small institutions providing moral treatment into the large and unwieldy state hospitals of the late nineteenth century has been well documented (Grob 1966, 1983; Scull, 1979, 1984). Despite efforts of reformers, these institutions remained intractably resistant to change until, in the mid-twentieth century, they began to empty out in the movement known as deinstitutionalization. As one nineteenth century asylum doctor put it, the asylum was like a convenient lumber room that, once available, invariably filled to overflowing with lumber. "Friends are only too willing, in their poverty, to place away the human encumbrance of the family at county expense" (Scull 1979:253).[3]

The move to empty institutions that followed on Kennedy's proposal radically changed the landscape in which psychiatric patients found themselves.[4] It has resulted in institutions like the Douglass Center, with its inner-city location and ideology of community care, and in the other kinds of facilities—outpatient centers, boarding homes, and halfway houses—that were mentioned in chapter 2. We have already seen that the results of this movement are problematic. The medications developed in the 1950s and often credited with making community care possible may alleviate some of the symptoms that bring patients to the hospital but do not resolve issues of chronicity and dependence. The provision of care outside institutions is often inadequate to address the magnitude of patients' problems, and some community-based care has replicated conditions in the state hospitals it is intended to replace (Estroff 1981, 1985). Patients "fall between the cracks" of the new system in ways that parallel their abandonment to the "warehouses" of the old system (Segal et al. 1977). Though no one advocates returning to the asylums of the past, criticism of deinstitutionalization has become widespread. One historian of psychiatry asks rather plaintively, "If it is wrong to get patients out of the mental hospital, and wrong to keep them in, what are we to do with them?" (Jones 1982:221).

Recent historians of psychiatry have engaged in an intense and sometimes bitter debate about the background of the current controversy. For some, institutions are developed out of essentially humanitarian goals; when they fail, we must assume that human intentions are fallible and that social life as well as disease itself thwart even the best laid plans (e.g. Grob 1966, 1973, 1983). For others, institutions are developed out of mystifying ideologies that conceal their economic and political usefulness; in the case of the asylum, for example, the early institutions functioned to separate the mad from the working poor and to provide an environment in which psychiatry developed as a profession (Scull 1979).[5] Other writers are less involved with historical disputes than with the consequences of history; they raise questions about the nature of chronicity, the relationship between homelessness and mental illness, and the reasons for the underfunding of community treatment.[6]

Despite the great diversity of these perspectives, they tend to take shape around a series of related oppositions: idealism versus pragmatism, reform versus revision, hospital versus community, and humanitarianism versus economic interest. These oppositions are used as a theoretical vocabulary to frame the debate about how institutional psychiatry should be interpreted. At the same time they are the cultural common-sense terms in which the practice of psychiatry is described.[7] It is in this light that the history of the Douglass Center must be understood. The debate about whether deinstitutionalization is really a reform and about whether the community is the proper place for treatment exists inside the center in much the same terms as it does outside. The staff of the APU narrated a local history that expresses these themes and that leaves them unresolved for much the same reasons that more generalized accounts leave them unresolved. They echo Jones's question: what are we to do? But they echo it in a way that is thoroughly grounded in their own place and time. Their histories are expressive of a moment in which a larger movement of reform reverberated in the details of individual lives and particular institutions.

II

Those were the good old days!

—Sally Morrow

Kennedy's hopeful proposal set in motion a shift in public policy and funding patterns across the country. In 1966, three years after the enactment of the Community Mental Health Law, Midway City's Medical School and the state began a small mental health satellite, operated out of a trailer in one of the poor black neighborhoods of the city. Over the next few years other neighborhood centers were opened, and one of the psychiatric wards at the University was used as an emergency, short-term unit. Together this unit and the neighborhood centers formed an "Inner-City Community Mental Health Program."

The atmosphere of the neighborhood outpatient centers was informal. They were staffed by nurses, social workers, and "indigenous" (community) workers and were open to anyone who needed help. The staff did not dispense medication; difficult cases could be sent to the University or the state hospital.

Barbara, now the nurse chairperson on the APU, graduated from nursing school in 1964. She began working at the state hospital, but when the Community Mental Health Program began she left the hospital to work in one of the small neighborhood centers. She describes her work there:

> We had an open door policy at emergency services. A telephone call would come in about a crisis and we would go to them if they couldn't come, and go into the home. In one case the husband was sick in bed and wouldn't let his wife out of bed either! You had to laugh because of the very sadness of it. We couldn't get him out. There were many homes where people were ill; for instance there was a young college graduate who was not eating or sleeping and getting hostile. He talked with us very intellectually, denying that anything was wrong, refusing to admit a problem. The only solace for his family was to tell them they could call the police. At that time there was no emergency petition but the police would take people to the hospital out of empathy. We would use gentle coercion and family persuasion. We did a lot of counseling right on the spot. That was crisis intervention! You could talk to people right then about a problem. We got a call one evening from the police. A man was at a filling station. He was from the South, and everything he owned was in his car, and he had locked his keys in the car. He was very confused. They brought him over to the center. We kept him there and started tracing him, got a key made for his car, took him to a bank for money. We contacted his relatives but they wouldn't come. Finally one of the men at the filling station volunteered to drive him up to New York.
>
> We had a reputation—they knew we were there. We had a lot of homeless people, cases where we were like detectives. I felt more like a detective— finding shelter, driving people back and forth to missions.

Barbara emphasizes the mobility, egalitarian atmosphere, and hopefulness of this time. She was *right there* in the middle of people's lives, free to come and go when needed and to solve problems in whatever way possible. As Sally Morrow said about one of the neighborhood centers, "That was *my* idea of community mental health!" The staff of the centers were proud of their reputation in their neighborhoods; as Barbara put it, "I felt people should be helped outside state facilities. Without meds, we just talked to people to get them into hospitals."

Ben was not in a position to express this kind of unself-conscious nostalgia; the early period of community mental health coincided with his days in medical school and an innocence he now feels he has lost. He described his initial involvement with his characteristic blending of cynicism and wistfulness:

> When I was a medical student [at the University] they talked about the integration of medicine and the community. I had my psycho-social period then; I worked at Sears and lived in a hovel. I used to walk through our [present]

catchment area to work. It whetted my appetite for community medicine. I
like seedy places. My contempt for the establishment was incredible. I was
interested in connection *to the community.*[8]

In a revealing mixing of categories, Ben equates the community he
walked through as a medical student with the present catchment area,
thus conflating a notion of human connection with the bureaucratic
device that orders the population of the city according to institutional
requirements. For him the community of which Barbara still speaks so
confidently has been layered over by an administrative convention,
paralleling his sardonic distancing from his earlier contempt for institutional authority.

In the late sixties and early seventies, as the state began to carry out
the policy of deinstitutionalization, it became harder to send the more
difficult cases to the state hospital. It was clear that the University would
not be able to care for the large numbers of patients, many without insurance, who were being released into the area from the hospital, nor
for the new patients who could no longer be sent there. The directors
of the Inner-City Program began, as Giuliani put it, "to think of a building." It was financially and politically a good time to draw on the state's
willingness to back new projects in community mental health. And, as
one University planner put it, "I also thought a financial crunch was
coming and that we would only survive by linking up with the state. . . . I
wanted the center to take care of bread-and-butter psycho-social rescue
work, leaving the University free to develop as a tertiary care center."

The Douglass Center was to provide short-term care, keeping patients out of the hospital as much as possible. Younger patients who had
never suffered long-term hospitalization would be treated quickly and
kept in contact with their families and neighborhoods so that they would
not become dependent on institutional care; the link to University-based
psychiatry would result in better care than in the isolated state hospitals.
The hospital would have a swimming pool and auditorium that would
attract community participation; it would function like a shopping mall
to enliven the surrounding urban blight. It would be, in Ben's words,
"An oasis of mental health, with indigenous workers like Trina who
would know more about community folks." The wide-open front door
was to be symbolic of the center's openness to its neighbors.

The emergency wing of the Douglass Center was initially intended
to provide what Ben called a "crash pad," a place where people in crisis
could be treated quickly—without inducting them into an institutional
setting—and returned to their lives in the community. This way of responding to emergencies developed in the late sixties and early seventies
and combined several approaches that had not been formally associated
until then. The unit would be like a general hospital emergency ward

in its twenty-four-hour service, acceptance of walk-in patients, and attention to all referrals. The treatment offered, particularly psychotropic medication, would come from psychiatry. The team approach to treatment, an ideology of crisis intervention, and a strong reliance on the telephone had been developed by the community mental health movement.[9] This assemblage of hitherto separate kinds of treatment aimed to keep the hospital open to its environment and to prevent patients from long-term dependence. Ben described the rationale as a combination of deinstitutionalization and prevention.

> The object in the 1960s was preventative mental health services, indigenous services. These would deal with a different stream of people from those who were deinstitutionalized; we would provide a refuge, keeping people on the street and out of the state hospital.

III

> Then what happened? It was an overpromise but such a nice one.
>
> —BEN CALDWELL

A big architectural firm was hired to plan the building. But political changes caused the mental health department to lose its support at the state level and so work on the building was delayed. Local interest groups and the press drew attention to the issue; in the neighborhood, community leaders organized demonstrations in support of the center and, eventually, the project was resumed. Work began on the building. But by that time costs had gone up; there was no money for the swimming pool or the extras that had been planned as attractions for the neighborhood. As Anthony Giuliani described it:

> This building reflects the change in budget; it was supposed to be taller, with no closed spaces inside and the community free to walk in and out; wards were designed to resemble neighborhood houses. Budget changes and a change in architect firms changed that and the old ideas about community participation got lost in the struggle.

When the building was completed at last, one of the University planners describes his disappointment.

> I went through the building once before the patients came. It was a disappointment. It didn't have the warmth [we had planned]; it was like a mental hospital.

Thus the center emerged out of an ideal that was, in fact, more real to the indigenous workers and residents with their dreams of community than it was to the University and the state, which used it to solve the practical problem of nonpaying patients. Fed by a contradictory mix of contemporary theory and University needs, the center was diminished and, quite literally, "shortened" by the time the structure was finally in place. The architectual conventions of institutionalization prevailed over the ideal of warmth.

For a while, despite the link to the University, the center was a stepchild, slow to develop. Giuliani was hired as director of inpatient services and began to staff the inpatient wards. Emergency Services was the first to open; the APU was the first inpatient unit, handling emergencies while the rest of the building remained empty. The unit was staffed by the same people who worked in the old community centers. Barbara said, "When the news came we were moving we were all in mourning." For them, the work was far less attractive than what they used to do. As Sally put it, "When we moved we became a hospital." Barbara describes the change in roles that this entailed:

> We had to reprogram ourselves to an inpatient model, had to change our ways of thinking; it was different for all of us. It wasn't so hard for the nurses because we had had it (hospital training) once, but the others (mental health workers) found it hard. We taught them how to do blood pressures, make beds. Everyone was answering the telephone. As time went on we began to define our roles differently.

The new definition of the situation did not come from these workers, but from the administrative changes that made the unit, increasingly, a bureaucratic entity. Ben Caldwell was hired to organize Emergency Services and run the APU. Coming into an entirely new and unformed situation, he was prepared to take risks to organize it to fit his own ideas. He responded to the undifferentiated roles of the original staff members by establishing a new distribution of power:

> The staff said, like hell we're going to be on an inpatient ward; we're supposed to drive around looking for psychotics. Also, there was a problem of who was in charge, me or the nurse. At first I didn't care. Then I passed my boards and came back so grandiose and took the nurse into her office and screamed at her and said she wasn't going to run it. (I couldn't believe I'd done it, it must have been the fulfillment of some sort of Oedipal rage. I went home and said, well, I can always get another job.) We had a meeting—I've always been a test case—and the nurse was hurt. I rearranged office space and she left.

Ben falls back on a parenthetical psychoanalytic explanation, but in fact his rearrangement of the hierarchy was in harmony with the institutional nature—the "office space"—of the unit; he tested the situation to see whether he could contain a staff that had become accustomed to defining their own terms of work.[10]

The mental health workers, too, had to change their positions, not only geographically, but in relation to their coworkers. As Ben continued:

> We also had the notion of the indigenous worker. Trina was one of the originals. We didn't realize they might be nuts. Now they're colonized; she's just a regular hospital employee.

We have seen that this way of looking at the indigenous workers continued to be a theme on the unit. They were "just hospital employees," bureaucratized and set to the mindless processing of patients; at the same time they were unable to rise above the history of their link to the patients' world.

As the number of patients increased, Ben found that he had to get some help. A year after the unit opened, he asked for a resident. This was when he first threatened to quit: "I've had to quit so many times to get things." The next year, he "quit" again and Sam was hired to direct the inpatient unit. During these early years, Ben discovered an effective way to deal with the paradoxes of the work, a way which colored the unit's operation from then on:

> One of the first residents said it wouldn't work. That's when I developed my administrative style. I said, Well, I'll do it. Please don't do anything that violates your ethical, moral code. Give it to me and I'll do it.

Ben also discovered that there was a nice fit between his sardonic style and the difficulty of the work, and he learned, as time went on, the fun of expressing pleasure in this. "When I took this job," he said, "it sounded terrible. My God, I thought, this would be so bad you couldn't fail!" With this attitude, he put together the unit's "on the ground" compromise between the original grassroots orientation and the reality of operating within a large institution.

IV

> When they finally got it open . . . there was the question of how to make it work.
>
> —BEN CALDWELL

The staff were agreed that as the building filled up with inpatient services it became, as Sally said, more of a hospital. Reaching a certain critical mass changed its character. Anthony Giuliani felt that "There's a point at which one more inpatient unit causes a much higher level of complexity, a point where a change in quantity causes a change in quality . . . There has been a gradual development in the volume of services, the complexity of the institution, and the interrelationship with other institutions."

These changes affected the way the nurses and mental health workers experienced their work. Sally described the difference, speaking from her position as screening nurse:

> *Now if we got someone in here [whose situation needed sorting out] we would be more limited [than in the community center days]; we have to deal with the psychiatric side of it. Now if someone wants us to go to their home we can't . . . I feel disappointed; I miss the outreach and the home visits.*

> *Growth seems to have come from our accessibility. People needed it before but somehow they managed. Now everything is so accessible, some of them come in off the street and make up things. They say "I need help" and you have to drag out of them what they need. Also the police and other agencies are more aware of the Douglass Center. The whole city thinks we should be all things to all people.*

> *The paperwork has increased, of course. And of course in the old days we didn't have medication to dispense. Most of the patients were in real crisis; we dealt with it by intervening, talking, brief therapy, and sending them to clinics. Now medicine is more accessible. But very often medication is not always indicated. Some of the residents rely on the prescription pad.*

> *I don't believe we were giving as many meds on the Unit then, we didn't pump them full of crappy meds. We use more now, because of the physicians and because patients are staying longer. And they are ordering all sorts of tests and that shit. Now they use all the medical clinics over at the University [e.g., for tests on patients]. A person can have dental caries all their life and come to the Douglass Center and get a whole new set of teeth!*

The center threatened to fill up; its very existence suggested a promise that the staff could not keep. Sally suggests that to some extent medication filled this gap, making up for the time and energy that was once available when the staff had mobility and less paperwork. But the very fact of giving medication implies that this institution—a hospital—provides *medicine,* and medicine potentially encompasses the whole body, even the teeth. The limits to what the hospital can provide are not clear. Bea Radnor mentioned this in a conversation about Sam's early days on the unit, when he was trying to learn the contours of the job:

There are multiple problems here (in the hospital)—like malnutrition. Sam was very sensitive to this, not certain where to draw the line . . . it's not easy for me, either, but I have to follow the guidelines. The state is paying for psychiatric *treatment.*

Sally's complaint is that no amount of "guidelines" can counteract the effect of the hospital environment on the expectations of the staff or the patients.[11]

The staff describe a transitional period, the "early days" of the center, when the unit still retained a rather open, casual character. The staff sometimes took the patients out on day-trips in the city and some patients ate their meals upstairs in the cafeteria.[12] But this flexibility diminished as the unit's role became more defined and the hospital's organization more complex and hierarchical. Robert Naumann described it as a "gradual adding of layers, with the key positions going to MDs." Greater restriction on the movement of both the staff and the patients had its most obvious effect on the mental health workers, who found themselves deprived of the role they had once had. Paul spoke bitterly of this:

I used to do things for the patients [during the early days of the unit's existence], like playing guitar, getting cigarettes for them, singing. But since we got no recognition for it, we stopped. Now the patients don't get nothing *but a bed and three lousy meals. We used to have a staff lounge but now we have no place to get away from the patients. We're supposed to be back here all day long. The other staff don't have to do anything except sit at a desk, it's easy to escape when you're at a desk. We're stuck back here. And I'm not saying it [the patient's craziness] don't rub off. You have to learn to protect yourself. You tune out. You just do what you have to do and what is benevolent for the patients and then think about something else. I think of this as a stop on the way to another job.*

These accounts by the staff members reflect their position in relation to the period before the APU developed its present form. Sally, Barbara, and Paul experienced their roles in the hospital as profoundly different from what was expected from them as community workers. Barbara has become an administrator, relatively removed from patients; Sally gives medicine; and Paul takes a bitter, do-nothing approach to his custodial duties. They see the development of the hospital in terms of changes that rendered them both more and less responsible for patients. There seem to be more patients and their needs are more overwhelming, but the patients are handled in an impersonal, efficient style that makes the old kind of involvement impossible. The work of connecting the patients to the community has become desk work and telephone work, assigned to a growing intermediate level of nurses, social workers, and students.

For the staff who are higher up in the hierarchy, these changes disappointed, but they also opened up new possibilities. While some of the original planners simply turned their attention elsewhere, for Ben, and later Sam, the unit was a newly formed, malleable environment where they could try out ideas and develop a personal and administrative style. Ben no longer believed that the community psychiatry envisioned by the early planners of the Center was possible.

> *[In community psychiatry] we thought, all we have to do is . . . whatever, a la Goffman, Laing. [Now] I can sit back and be puzzled why it doesn't work. That's the fascinating part. Not to negate Giuliani's humanitarianism, but it's more complicated than that.*

Ben suggests that the very fact that he no longer knows where the work is going has become its justification. "I want to be [here] in case something happens. Who knows what will happen in psychiatry!"[13]

One of the original planners of the Douglass Center told me that "Social institutions are like coral reefs, built out of the skeletons of what was once there." We can see the truth of this in the layered history described by the APU staff, in which both the state hospital and an earlier phase of community psychiatry underlie current practice. At the same time, the staff's narratives remind us that this layering is no simple progression: theirs is not a single history but a chorus of voices reflecting different positions in relation to shifting, sometimes contradictory, views of the past. They also remind us that the visual metaphor of a "view" or "perspective" on the past fails to capture the emotion with which it is imbued; nostalgia, disappointment, pride, anger, and confusion are all present in these narratives and bring past feeling into present practice.

These narratives suggest a continuity between the current contradictions experienced by the staff and the history of psychiatry itself. The staff mix institutonal, community, and everyday language in ways that suggest that none of these vocabularies provides a cohesive or satisfactory way of talking about what they do. And they provide metaphors that suggest the ambiguities inherent in the history they have inherited. Thus, for example, Ben's metaphor of the mall suggests that the hospital supplies a product (products?) that the neighborhood might find desirable; his comparison to an oasis implies a retreat and place of abundance in the midst of a desert. The contradictory implications of these metaphors are realized in the public's apparently insatiable demand for more, and more extensive, care, and its tendency to use the center as a haven or a source of goods (witness the barred front door).

The staff's accounts of their history are pervaded by the theme of unforeseen consequences: the modification of fantasy by events. Spoken from a position of embeddedness in practice, they express at once an awareness of the ongoingness of contradiction and of the necessity for pragmatism in the face of human, and institutional, frailty.

FIVE

Whatever Takes Less Writing

I

He's not mentally ill, he's just an ass!

—Duane Powers

Diagnosis was central to the activities of the APU but, at the same time, peripheral to its major purpose. On the one hand, patients became patients by virtue of being diagnosed with a psychiatric illness and their diagnosis sometimes contributed to decisions about disposition; on the other hand, diagnosis was malleable and ambiguous, often valued more for its strategic than its medical purposes. One of the main tasks of students on the APU was to learn how to diagnose, what purposes to use diagnoses for, and when to ignore or resist a diagnosis.

On Emergency Services, diagnosis was usually accomplished either before a patient arrived (the patient "carried" a diagnosis already) or as a result of an examination in Screening, where residents learned to apply a fairly small number of psychiatric diagnoses to the large number of people passing through their hands. This process required the development of interviewing skills, familiarity with diagnostic categories, and sometimes an awareness of psychodynamic principles.[1] Residents also learned the use of psychiatric medications as part of the process of diagnosis, quickly becoming accustomed to the standard medicines and dosages.

The main resource for the practice of diagnosis on Emergency Services was the *Diagnostic and Statistical Manual of Mental Disorders, Third Edition* (APA 1980). "DSM III," as it is called, is a large volume in which all the psychiatric disorders are given in encyclopedic form, each with its typical features, age at onset, and course; decision trees are provided to aid in differential diagnosis.[2] A tattered copy was attached with a chain to the resident's desk in screening (in Walter's drawing it can be seen as "vital to the work") and consulted frequently by residents and medical students as they attempted to match patients' symptoms with the available categories. Patients who came in "carrying" a diagnosis from a past admission had to be evaluated; patients who came in for the first time had to be given some kind of label (even if only the label "deferred diagnosis"). Patients could not be admitted unless a number corresponding to a category in DSM III had been entered on their charts.

Students quickly learned to translate specific behaviors into the language of psychiatry: "the patient talks very fast" became "pressured speech" and "the patient doesn't make any sense" became "flight of ideas" or "loose associations." Typical patterns or clusters of such behaviors could then be recognized as pointing to the specific disorders described in DSM III.[3] Here, for example, is part of the DSM III description of schizophrenia: "The major disturbance in the content of thought involves delusions that are often multiple, fragmented or bizarre . . . certain delusions are far more common in this disorder than in other psychiatric disorders" (1980:182). To discover the "content" of a patient's thought, residents used psychiatric interviewing techniques, asking both direct and indirect questions designed to elicit delusions, suicidal thoughts, and unusual uses of language. These techniques treat the patient's personality as a field of signs and symptoms penetrable by the gaze of the physician; the diagnosis provides an "agreed label that essentializes the patient" (Light 1980:194).

The residents and medical students who worked in Emergency Services considered it a good place to learn diagnosis because they were able to see a great variety of patients. One medical student said of his rotation, "I got to see a lot of things my classmates didn't see. For instance, manic-depression; my classmates saw one or two cases, I saw dozens." This experience enabled students to feel competent at diagnosis and therefore, as one student put it, "independent."[4] One student described passing from an initial nervousness ("When someone asked me if I wanted a patient to interview, I'd say no") to an increasing sense of competence. Within a couple of weeks on the unit he said, "By this point I've got the standard diagnoses down—schizophrenia, depression, classic features. I can tell you what to do."

This kind of confidence came in part from a sense of having had enough patients to practice on: one student said "I saw so much florid psychosis and I learned so much medicine." It also came from experiences of patients' behavior that seemed to match that described for their diagnoses. For example, when patients responded to particular medications (such as lithium for manic-depression) this tended to confirm the diagnosis that had suggested the medication in the first place. A patient's angry or passive response to being interviewed could also suggest the accuracy of the diagnosis, a process Goffman called "looping" (1961).

However, this sense of "learning medicine" and belief in the objective validity of diagnosis was constantly undermined by many of the situations students faced. The student who felt, initially, that he "could tell you what to do," said a week later that he had realized that, "You couldn't make a mistake down here." He realized that the freedom given him to practice suggested that whatever he did would make no difference. By the end of his rotation on the unit he commented that "Treatment is beginning to seem pretty arbitrary to me." While he was expected to master the techniques of psychiatric diagnosis, he was also exposed to many situations in which the unit thwarted, undermined, or played with those same techniques. For example, a student asked Sam, following an interview with a patient, "Do you think he's schizophrenic?" Sam said, "I thought he was psychotic, but what kind I'm not sure. Well, if Mellaril or Haldol works, use it. 'If it works, shoot with a broom.'" Sam undoes any notion of a neat relationship between diagnosis and medicine, yet leaves open the possibility that someone can eventually figure out what kind of psychotic the patient is. Thus the student had to learn that diagnosis was true, useful, *and* tentative, even meaningless.

One way the more experienced staff taught students to question diagnosis was to highlight the process of charting. The patient's chart could be seen as an entity with a life of its own,[5] with diagnosis as an essential feature *of the chart* but not necessarily of the patient. In this conversation, for example, Sam was discussing the presentation of an involuntary patient at a hearing to determine whether he would be retained.

SAM: At the hearing you have to establish that he's mentally ill . . . has a bipolar affective disorder.

STUDENT: We have him as schizophrenic.

SAM: Those are just details. Put whatever you like, whatever takes less writing.

The point was to get the patient committed as efficiently as possible; the task of the moment was to establish his illness, but the exact diagnosis was irrelevant. Sam described this recognition of the separation between the patient and the diagnosis as one of the things that marked his assimilation into the culture of the unit.

I stopped paying attention to diagnosis and would put down the previous one [already in the chart]. I remember the resident liked debating it but I didn't give a damn . . . unaccountably I lost interest.

One reason for this loss of interest was that very often the problem of diagnosis could be passed on to the next person in line. The usefulness of diagnosis could thus be maintained as an ideal while in practice considered peripheral to the needs of the unit. Patients were on the unit such a short time that the decision did not need to be made there, and the more experienced staff recognized that the students' interest in "debating it" was the result of their own desire to become competent clinicians. Sometimes this disjunction between the unit's and the student's interests was made very explicit.

■ Duane says of a new patient that he doesn't know whether she's schizophrenic or manic. He says to Sam, "What do you think?"

SAM: Well, let me ask another. First, does she need more than a week of treatment?

DUANE: She's been on Haldol and there's absolutely no change in three days.

[They discuss whether switching to Mellaril would make a difference.]

SAM: How about we transfer her to her catchment area hospital? Work on that . . . as to whether she's manic, I may not have time to look at her before she leaves but my opinion probably has less to do with what happens than that of the next person. Write on the chart that you recommend looking at the question of manic-depression.

DUANE: Your opinion is valuable to *me.*

SAM: Well, I'll take a look at her for *you,* not for the patient.

The patient's lack of response to medication suggests that the diagnosis is incorrect. Duane wants to discover what features of the patient's behavior might lead Sam to conclude that she is, in fact, manic. But while Sam recognizes that the diagnosis will eventually be important to treatment of the patient, he feels that attention to it is not an efficient use of his time on the unit; the problem can be handled in the chart.

In the following discussion we see both an explicit teaching of diagnostic skill and a demonstration that the local situation required referring the final decision to another facility. The attending psychiatrist from the University was working on Screening, helping a resident and a medical student decide whether to admit a new patient. The patient was a recent immigrant from Puerto Rico who had daily episodes of sudden anger in which he became violent.

■   The resident describes the patient as neatly dressed, with no phobias, delusions, or suicidal ideation, with coherent thought and appropriate affect.

PSYCHIATRIST [to medical student]: Well, what do you think?

MEDICAL STUDENT: Personality disorder.

PSYCHIATRIST: Why? I didn't hear anything so far . . .

RESIDENT: I wouldn't call him that.

PSYCHIATRIST: This is not a long-term maladaptive problem; he functions well, has skills, is married.

MEDICAL STUDENT: Intermittent explosive disorder?

PSYCHIATRIST: What do you know about it? The concept is that he becomes explosive out of character but is not angry between episodes. But this doesn't fit. Anyway, this diagnosis won't exist in DSM IV. It doesn't fit. What else remains?

RESIDENT: He probably drinks much more than he will admit and is dealing with prejudice and isolation [as an immigrant]. "Adjustment disorder" with associated alcohol abuse.

PSYCHIATRIST TO STUDENT: You see how you approach this fellow; you get all the information, rule out [some] possibilities, and ask, do the symptoms fit the diagnostic possibilities? If the medical model is not that helpful you can go for "disorder" (the insurance will still pay).

RESIDENT: I'm more comfortable with a deferred diagnosis.

PSYCHIATRIST: How can you help him?

[They discuss outpatient therapy, alcohol counseling. The resident explains that he didn't hospitalize the patient because he has a job, a wife who feels comfortable taking him home, and he is intelligent.]

The psychiatrist teaches the students to try to gather "all the information," some of which, as in the case of alcohol consumption, may be hidden. Once they have it (he assumes enough for a preliminary decision will be available in this short interview) they look for an approximate fit between the patient's symptoms and the available diagnostic categories. The psychiatrist suggests that the medical model may not work (there may not be an identifiable disease) but that "disorders" are available to describe less specific conditions still covered by insurance.

He lets them know that DSM III itself can be arbitrary; he sees the diagnosis proposed by the student as so useless that it will be eliminated from a fourth edition. Finally, though the emphasis in much of the discussion is pathology (even in the initial report which lists what the patient doesn't have)[6] the outcome of the session is a result of connecting the diagnostic categories with practical considerations about where to send the patient.

In these discussions, diagnosis is presented as a process of matching available categories with "facts" or "information" about the patient. Sometimes, however, psychiatrists introduced another layer of complexity into the process, using the analytic perspective that was important at the University. Despite the fact the psychoanalysis was rarely considered directly relevant on Emergency Services, psychodynamic interpretations, even in rather fragmentary form, sometimes gave a feeling of depth to discussions of diagnosis. This was especially the case in comments that gave primacy to the underlying emotional tone of a diagnostic label. For instance, one day the attending psychiatrist on Screening interviewed a suicidal young man. The man expressed embarrassment at his botched suicide attempt, to which the attending replied, "You're more tormented than crazy." In the immediate discussion of what to do with this patient, the psychiatrist simply addressed his depression, his need for medication, and the necessity of hospitalization due to suicide risk. But later, in an almost casual aside, he said, "The guy's borderline; he'll *always* be tormented." Despite an appearance of craziness (in this case a synonym for "psychotic") the underlying and unresolvable issue is, in his view, the "torment" of the borderline patient.[7]

The way psychodynamic interpretation involves "feeling the diagnosis" has been discussed effectively by Light, who points out that "a great deal of 'feel' is evident in how diagnoses are made . . . residents learn how to 'feel' while still appearing professionally precise." Interpretations and decisions based on "feel" have behind them the "theoretical machinery" of psychodynamic theory, particularly the idea of countertransference (1980:181–182).

■ A new medical student was very excited after seeing an attending from the university interview a patient on screening. He reported that Dr. B said, "I think he has psychiatric problems but they are not acute." Then Dr. B turned to the patient and said, "You haven't proved to me that you're crazy." The patient asked, "How do I prove it?" Dr. B said, "You just are if you are."[8] He invited the patient to stay for the discussion, then asked the residents for opinions. One thought the patient was psychotic, another, that organicity should be ruled out. Dr. B agreed with everyone, saying that all their ideas were possible. Dr. B then made a decision to send him back to the clinic he had come from. At this point the patient started talking about medicines in an anxious, rambling way. Suddenly, Dr. B stopped him and said "I am feeling exasperated because *he* is feeling exasperated. If he's that exasperated, we should admit him." The student was fascinated by this willingness of the older doctor to trust his countertransference. He said, "Here's a guy who intellectually would have sent the guy back out on the streets but he made an important judgment on the basis of emotions and then rationalized it. I was also exasperated but I wouldn't have known what to do; this is what separates the average shrink from the good shrink."

Thus, while the need for efficiency precluded much theoretical elaboration, the APU and Screening offered brief opportunities for the experienced, psychoanalytically inclined staff to demonstrate "being a good shrink" by showing the students that the diagnostic categories could be related to their own feelings about patients. In the following passage another student describes a similar episode, one that made him realize his diagnostic powers were still limited.

> But if you get a patient like I had yesterday . . . ! I thought she was paranoid personality disorder. Everything she said wasn't delusional. Dave [a resident] guessed bipolar affective. But Dr. B said my patient was paranoid schizophrenic on the basis that she knew him better than he knew himself. My patient would sense Dr. B's intentions . . . Dr. B says it's his clinical knowledge, not in the books.

The student wants to exclude that part of the patient's behavior that seemed normal to him, but Dr. B's "clinical knowledge" allows him to see the patient "whole" (all of a piece with her diagnosis) through the effect she has on him. Dr. B is also indicating that the student must make his decisions "in action" rather than "from the book," that the diagnostic categories "as written" cannot be relied on in practice.

We saw in earlier discussions of diagnosis that this kind of psychoanalytic orientation could be a kind of luxury, indulged in when there was time. Often, the point made to students was that although diagnosis might be fun to talk about their task was to stay oriented to the immediate context. Diagnosis had either to be used to get the patient out, or it had to be set aside so that other factors could be attended to. One way to use diagnosis was to use it strategically in accordance with the opportunities for placement that might be available. We saw this in the case of the Judge. The actual diagnosis carried by Judge when he entered the unit had nothing to do with how he was treated, but the diagnoses that the staff experimented with were intended to help him match a placement. Another use of diagnosis, also evident in the case of Judge, was to distinguish patients belonging to the APU from those that could be passed on to others. Sometimes the attempt to secure a passage to a different facility resulted in a territorial battle, as in the case of a struggle over the question of whether a patient was competent to stand trial. The staff were motivated to pass on those problems they felt were not "normal" for the unit; florid psychosis and violence, for example, were considered problems for which the unit could find fairly quick resolutions, whereas sociopathic behavior, senile dementia, and the problems of adolescents were not.[9] In these cases it was in the interest of the unit to emphasize that the patient's diagnosis made him unsuited to their care. Here is a discussion in which the central issue is the patient's unsuitability to the unit.

■ A patient was brought from jail after having been arrested for beating his wife. He had a history of drug and alcohol abuse and a diagnosis of "antisocial personality." One of the satellite mental health centers had "persuaded the judge" to refer him to the APU, "sneaking him in," in Robert's view because they "imagine that he is salvageable." The medical student expressed confusion about what to do since there seemed to be a choice between "jail" and "commitment," with pressure from outside for commitment. Through all of this discussion Ronnie chanted "Jail! Jail! He's *criminal*, not mental. He's dangerous, not crazy!"

At times the staff taught students to ignore or work around diagnosis, to pay attention primarily to the immediate situation of the patient. Here, for instance, a student learns that a practical matter important to the patient may in fact be the most crucial factor in her treatment. The patient had been brought in by the police for shouting at city hall.

STUDENT: She says this is the best place she's ever been.

SAM: Find out about her shouting. Does she think it was reasonable? Her complaint may be legitimate. Maybe she could find other avenues . . .

On another occasion, Sam used a recent article to legitimize the pragmatic orientation of the unit:

SAM [to a resident]: I don't think we can offer traditional psychotherapy here; patients need a concrete reality approach. This patient's problem is housing and he *says* that's his problem. In this article [which he had just handed out] Bullock, who's an analyst, comes near what we're trying; he proposes a time-frame [that is, short-term intervention] consistent with ours.

Thus students were taught to approach problems with the question "What is needed in this context?" The staff called this "flexibility." Barbara expressed admiration for Ben's ability to recognize this trait when he hired new people: "Flexibility," she said "is important to our make-up as a unit." To be successful on the unit, the staff had to be "down to earth" and "point-blank" in dealing with patients and with each other.

They had to assume that the usefulness of psychiatric categories was always contingent on the immediate situation. Sam said about the teaching of students:

> *This is like sending soldiers into a mock battle. They think they've lost but really the purpose was to test something else, like whether their boots were waterproof. You think you're operating under one model and it turns out to be something else.*

One way the staff expressed "something else" was to give patients labels that fit their relationship to the unit. These labels were produced in somewhat the same way as diagnostic categories but the "essential" traits were those that predicted the patient's place in the mental health system. This is the process we saw in the case of Judge: the gradual institution of a local label—"pet"—which described him more accurately in relation to the unit than "organic brain syndrome." This description summarized his characteristic stance—one could almost say his temperament—and entailed a certain vision of how he should be treated.

Other local labels described the resilience of the patient. One category was "tough." Nolan, the patient who thought she was God, was tough because, despite her illness, she seemed unlikely to be harmed by the environment. As Ben put it, "Some patients are tough and resilient regardless of how crazy they are. No one was worried at the idea of Nolan loose in the Port Authority. She fit there." On the other hand "vulnerable" patients (for example, teenage girls) could be harmed by the unit and had to be quickly moved to a safer environment. Sam said:

> *The real mental status exam is "Is this patient breakable?" If so, the staff come to me and say, "Come here, there's a breakable patient who doesn't belong here." This is a gut feeling; we feel the discordance between the patient and the surroundings.*

Perhaps the most common local label was "repeater." Some patients were "despised repeaters," like King James with his intense determination to get back onto the unit. Sam described King James as "horribly antagonistic, disgusting . . . He would whine and elicit dislike; we would provide that [that is, dislike] for him and in that sense, we were reliable for him." "Beloved repeaters," on the other hand, were patients who were not impulsive or suicidal (thus, did not require a great deal of watching) and who had "a certain quality of enjoyment." They could "be glad to see us, and ask for maintenance and be comforted." We will look more closely at these patients in the next chapter; here, the point is that the formal diagnostic system was paralleled by one that reflected areas of local practice that warranted certain kinds of predictive labeling. Such categories were not applied very systematically; many patients were in and out too fast to merit a homemade designation, but by applying them to difficult or outstanding patients, the staff created a local language that indicated whether a patient needed a room near the nurses' station or could survive on a bus to New York.[10]

Those who did not grasp the implicit, tacit, and local aspects of diagnosis and insisted on a single interpretation or a single source (such as DSM III or psychoanalytic theory) failed to grasp the essence of practice on the unit. As Sam said of a nurse who was on the unit a very short time, "She knew all the rules but she was totally useless."

II

The Other, as object of knowledge, must be separate, distinct and preferably distant from the knower.

—JOHANNES FABIAN (1983:121)

The farther you get from patients (the more) you can show you're an empathic person but the closer you are the less you can be good.

—BEN CALDWELL

The asylum . . . organized [guilt] for the madman as a consciousness of himself, and as a non-reciprocal relation to the keeper; it organized it for the man of reason as an awareness of the Other . . .

—MICHEL FOUCAULT (1973:147)

We have seen that "deep" diagnosis, and particularly the use of psychodynamic interpretations of the clinician's feelings, sometimes appeared in a rather fragmented way even in routine screening interviews. But there was another use for this kind of diagnosis, one that touched on a central problem of work on the APU. The APU staff had to learn how to keep an emotional distance from patients, how to deal with the complex relationship between "empathy," "closeness," and "goodness" that is summed up in Ben's comment above. Diagnosis played a dual part in this learning, serving to objectify both the patient and the feelings of the clinician for the patient.[11]

A student on the unit soon came up against the difficult implications of his acquisition of knowledge about a patient. In this example a student talks about his reaction after sending a patient to a locked ward at the VA hospital. The student has prepared his case for a hearing in which the patient was presented as potentially homicidal.

The thing that's striking me today is the enormity of what happened at that hearing. I'm primarily responsible for sending this man somewhere he doesn't want to go and can't get out of. Supposedly it's in his best interests but I don't really know. It's in the interest of the system. Even if I didn't do it someone else would have but still, I did it. It's not while you're doing it [that you notice] because Wishinski is standing there saying this is what should be done . . . If I'd really wanted to sabotage the decision I could have. I didn't have to tell them he's homicidal. I liked the guy and could have decided he deserved a chance. . . . He's really very kind, that's what makes it so hard. I'd make him my private patient if I had my degree.

The student was particularly disturbed by this because he wondered if his friendly style had been instrumental in extracting from the patient the very information that caused him to be retained.

I get pretty buddy-buddy with patients. I have trouble maintaining distance. I find I get a lot more from patients than Powers does. After a while [the patient described above] wouldn't talk to Powers anymore, but I was even able to talk to him about the VA.

Getting close to this patient demonstrated the uncomfortable association between power and knowledge; being good ("friendly") caused the patient to provide information that might have contributed to an outcome the patient didn't want. The student is unnerved to find himself an agent of "the system"; yet at the same time, the diagnosis helps him understand his decision in psychiatric terms.

Part of my ambivalence has to do with his disease. He got so much better because he was manic.[12] All his symptoms went away and it got down to dealing with a person with poor judgment. We're stuck with the books and his history.

In other words, is the patient's condition predictive, something ("his history") he is carrying with him that will cause him to act similarly again (according to "the books")? Or, has he become, on medication, simply "a person with poor judgment?" The student is torn between his feelings for a kind person with poor judgment and his knowledge that this is a psychiatric case with grave implications should the diagnosis prove predictive. All he can do is hope rather wistfully that he can be of more help "when he gets his degree."

This example points to the way diagnosis and feelings about a patient can intertwine. Part of the task of teaching on the unit was to show students how *not* to take the viewpoint of the patient.[13] This does not mean that the staff never responded empathetically to patients; as we will see in the next chapters the unit sometimes fostered acknowledgment of patients' perspectives. But efficient practice (in fact, any practice at all) required that staff create distance from patients and from their own feelings. The following example illustrates the relationship between the confinement of the patient, the issue of "perspective," and a student's struggle to come to terms with the power vested in her position.

Patients who were violent or disruptive were put into seclusion until they were quiet. As required by law, a patient in seclusion was checked at frequent intervals. Sometimes a patient who sensed himself going out of control would request seclusion. More often, the staff would matter-of-factly impose seclusion on a patient who appeared about to "escalate." Acutely psychotic patients often spent a period in seclusion until their medication began to take effect.

The use of seclusion sometimes shocked the medical students. Renee was a new medical student who had only been on the unit for a few days at the time of this incident. She was participating in a staffing meeting when a call came from the nurses' station to let Sam know that her patient, Mr. A, had been placed in seclusion after he was found to be hiding food in his room. He could be heard screaming and kicking at the door. Renee was obviously upset.

SAM [explaining the escalating noise]: This is a reaction to frustration.

RENEE: What do you expect? They [the patients] are always frustrated. No one goes to them when they come to the window. *I* would be frustrated.

ROBERT: Some of the patients get frustrated enough to find other ways to get what they need.

SAM: As a borderline he's good at inducing identification. You are identifying with him, and rightly so. The unit is more or less uniformly frustrating; when one person can put up with it and another loses it in ten minutes the distinction is diagnostically useful. Borderlines typically have trouble with this type of unit and this type of unit is good for them in providing limits.

[Renee is clearly disturbed and doesn't answer. The resident asks a question about a technical point in writing seclusion orders. Another call comes in, asking for an order for Haldol to calm Mr. A. The resident and Renee decide to go out and "say hello" to him before writing the order.]

This passage begins with Sam pointing matter-of-factly to the frustration-causing potential of the local environment. This is something that is taken for granted by the more experienced staff, but Renee reacts angrily, identifying with the patient's point of view. She assumes that the patient feels what she would feel, and she objects not only on his behalf but for all the patients. She is particularly disturbed by the window, where the patients look out but no one responds.

Robert reacts to her concern by suggesting that frustrating patients is, in fact, in their best interest because it stimulates them to try to get out of the unit. This was an important aspect of the local perspective, but when it seemed to make little impact on Renee, Sam broke in with a more clinical explanatory strategy. First, he says, her reaction to the patient *corresponds* to the patient's diagnosis. It is not part of *her* so much as it is one feature of what is wrong with the patient (he is "good at inducing identification"). Secondly, the frustration is not "in" the environment, but in the patient; she assumes that the patients feel as she would but in fact they feel in many different ways according to their condition. Her reaction (countertransference)[14] is an aspect of diagnosis, to be attended to as a sign of the patient's condition. Finally, the environment of the unit (uniformly frustrating as it is) can be redefined as "good" if the patient's needs are understood; he needs limits, which the unit is providing.

The resident and Renee come back from the seclusion room.

RENEE: He wouldn't calm down. We said, "We'll let you out in half an hour if you're calm." He's more violent locked up; he's afraid and he's claustrophobic.

SAM: I get the feeling we're all coming to believe we're brutes today. The patients are convincing us of our inhumanity.

RENEE: It *is* inhumane. Can you imagine being in there [she makes a gesture which takes in the whole "back" of the unit] without any windows?

WALTER: What would you learn from it?

RENEE: Not to get in, and not to tell anyone if you're suicidal.

SAM: Ironically, this is the unit you get *out* of the quickest. Some of what you say is accurate, but it *can* be a haven, or a Zen monastery, or a horrible prison. I'm glad you're talking about it; you're seeing it through the patient's eyes.

Renee makes it clear that her objection arises from seeing the situation through the patient's eyes—his fear, his inability to look out, his frustration at not being heard. Sam responds with a gesture of inclusion—"we *all* feel like brutes"—acknowledging that her feelings are shared, for the noise is clearly making everyone uncomfortable. Walter then tries to get Renee to use her "patient's" perspective to shift to a local interpretation (that she, if she were the patient, would learn not to behave in ways leading to hospitalization) but Renee instead offers her objection in terms of suicide risk (the patient's vulnerability). This objection was not addressed directly but was met by another attempt on Sam's part to show her a local understanding (that the unit was unusually easy to leave, actually less permanently confining than many) and to point out that any attempt to project a singular meaning onto the patients would eventually come up against the variety of their attitudes.

The meeting turns to the discussion of another patient, and Mr. A's shouting gradually subsides. Later, Sam turns back to Renee.

SAM: Now, let me tell you the inhumane direct solution to the treatment of Mr. A. What treatment does he need?

RENEE: He needs *everything,* a workup, everything [gesturing to her head] taken out and put back in!

SAM: He was depressed when he came in; now he's angry and we're depressed.

ROBERT: It's *safe* to be angry in here.

SAM: He's borderline. This means he's OK when he's not frustrated, but he can't be worked with. You put him in a confined space and he'll be angry and anxious. That is, he'll feel his own symptoms. How do you shoot a purple elephant? With a purple elephant gun. How do you shoot a white elephant? Hold his nose until he turns purple.

DUANE [to Renee]: You've got to understand that the *patient* is the one who is sick. Not you.

SAM: So you see we are doing precisely the right thing for this patient. He "dictates" for the resident to write on the seclusion order, "This poor patient, suffering from claustrophobia, was deprived of his rightful grape juice . . ."

ANOTHER RESIDENT: How about "grapes of wrath?"

DUANE [ironically]: I'm writing, "patient became agitated . . ."

This last conversation about Mr. A takes place after the sense of urgency created by his shouting has subsided. Renee, asked her opinion, says that the patient "needs everything taken out."[15] Implicit is the notion that everything, or anything, could be "fixed" with the right treatment; though Sam has asked her opinion, he ignores this innocent prescription. Instead, he suggests that the patient has "transferred" his depression to staff as his own anger has been liberated. Her emotion is, again, part of the patient. Robert then tries to persuade her to see the unit not as a prison but as a safe place for a particular kind of patient; suggesting a shift from a very generalized, true-for-everyone perspective to the more context-specific orientation of the unit. (The reader will recall that, in an earlier discussion about a different kind of patient, seclusion was rejected as inappropriate for his particular problem.) Sam then takes this argument a step further by showing that the treatment fits the patient's disorder; making him uncomfortable helps him by bringing his symptoms to the fore so that they can be dealt with. To "work with" a borderline, he has to be forced by the environment to change from a "white elephant" (depressed but unaware of it) to a "purple elephant" (angry and anxious). Duane steps in at this point with an attempt to reassure Renee that this coherence between the diagnosis and the patient's reaction to confinement is reassuring; the scary emotions are in the patient, not in her. The discussion ends with a joke that recognizes that the seclusion order is written to make the chart look good and does not necessarily reflect the local meaning of the situation.

In this episode the staff try to show Renee that there are two aspects to diagnosis that are useful for dealing with her feelings. The first is that diagnosis can be used to understand the patient's reactions as themselves diagnostic, not actually the same as the reactions she would have in the patient's shoes, but rather part of his problem. Secondly, Renee's own feelings become part of the diagnosis. This is a further elaboration of the point made in the first part of this chapter by the intuitive Dr. B. Dr. B has learned to treat his feelings as one indication of what the patient is feeling and therefore, as a sign that a particular diagnostic or disposition decision might be appropriate. Similarly in this case, Sam tries to locate Renee's reactions in the patient, whereas other staff members suggest that she be reassured by the psychological distance she can thereby achieve.

In his study of a psychoanalytically oriented institution, Light remarks that "the psychiatrist sees self as a scientific instrument. His feelings don't matter except as a presumed measure of the patient's feelings" (1980:174). While this orientation was not consistently expressed on the unit (and in fact there were other times when the feelings of staff mattered for their own sake) it was pressed into service when inexperienced clinicians found themselves unable to let go of "being good." In *Madness and Civilization* Foucault mentions that with the advent of moral treatment in the early nineteenth century the interior condition of the patient was brought into alignment with external conditions. "The patient [was] alienated in the psychiatrist" as his feelings became part of an interpretation based on reason (1973; Ingleby 1980:41). Similarly, in this conversation with Renee, the student's feelings are alienated in her teachers. Her feelings about the patient are used to make the patient's subjectivity into an object (borderline); thus the patient is something different from her and can be known as similar to others of his type.

This double alienation can be seen in the imagery of looking that pervades this exchange. Renee's identification with the patient leads her to see through the patient's eyes. The staff teach her that she should see the patient "objectively," as he "really" is (sick); she should see that his behavior points to his diagnosis. She is thus introduced to a psychiatric version of the clinical gaze that penetrates the patient and knows him through what he cannot know about himself. And she is urged to apply to herself (her own areas of unknowing) the same "informed vision" she brings to the patient.

When Mr. A was let out of seclusion a few hours after the discussion in staffing, he sneaked up behind Renee and grabbed her by the breasts. Walter said about this:

> *The* place *teaches . . .* we *could train a resident but we let them train themselves . . . They come around to our way eventually . . .*

The place taught partly because it pushed the student up against the patients in a way that made the learning of a new viewpoint a necessity. Just as Mr. A could teach himself through the unpleasantness of seclusion, Renee "trained herself" through immersion in a situation which, in Walter's view, induced the patient to act out his diagnosis in such a way that its truth became apparent.

The staff's discussion of Mr. A ended with a joke. The joke is not about the patient, or about Renee, but about the act of writing in the chart. The staff acknowledged that seclusion and the reasons for it had to be explained in language acceptable outside the unit ("agitation") while they expressed their own, mocking, version of what happened. This brings us to a closer look at another aspect of diagnosis on the APU, the staff's ambivalent relationship to charting.

III

What bothers me most is the paperwork.

—Duane Powers

The act of looking over and being looked over [is] a central means by which individuals are linked together in disciplinary space.

—Dreyfus and Rabinow (1982:156)

Have you ever tried to back a trailer into a driveway? The effect of what you do isn't what you thought it would be.

—SAM WISHINSKI

The ambiguous relationship between the chart and the patient's situation expressed in the joke about Mr. A's "rightful grape juice" points to a persistent tension on the unit. The staff were obliged to write about patients to accommodate the requirements of the state, the administration, and the law. This writing had to fit conventional forms and the standard vocabulary of psychiatric recordkeeping; it was perceived as one of the most time-consuming and burdensome aspects of work on the unit. The staff experienced a disjunction between what they wrote and what happened on the unit; sometimes, as we have seen, this disjunction could be articulated as strategy or made a source of humor. Sometimes it constituted the grounds for an outright resistance to "paperwork."

Patients' charts could be directly useful to staff. Often, a patient arrived at the clinic with a thick chart already in place (either at the Douglass Center itself or sent from elsewhere); this could be a rich source of information for staff and the basis for immediate decisions about a patient's treatment. For instance, a new patient was often given the type and dosage of medicine that had worked in the past. As we have seen, charts were also used to pass information to the next person involved with a patient. In the conversation given earlier about the patient that Sam had been willing to see for the sake of Duane's diagnostic curiosity, Sam suggests that by writing "look at manic-depression" in the chart, Duane can pass on his uncertainty to the next clinician in line, someone who can do something about it. This possibility of communicating with others through the chart could be comforting to staff, reassuring them that someone else would take up where they left off. Another aspect of the chart was its function as a legal document. Sam made it clear to students that it was legally necessary to be careful about what was written in patients' charts; an essential part of practice was "covering your ass" (making sure that the legal requirements were satisfied).

Like other aspects of treatment on the APU, however, the chart had to be handled efficiently. This was part of Sam's point when he told a student to put "whatever takes less writing." To deal efficiently with the chart, staff had to distinguish necessary writing—writing that would either make a difference to the patient or legally protect them—from writing that simply amplified the chart for its own sake. When diagnosis was an arbitary part of a patient's situation, for instance, it made no difference what went in the chart.

LILLIAN [about a patient's diagnosis]: Are you going with paranoid schizophrenic?

SAM: Yeah, might as well. It's the easiest and besides I know the [DSM III] number by heart.

Writing in the chart could also be used, very directly, to point to the difference between what happened on the unit and what was recorded for outside consumption.

■ It is the first meeting of the rotation and all the students are new. Sam gives them instructions on filling out the various forms, including the one for seclusion orders. He says, "Use some psychiatric euphemism for seclusion. 'Control' is never what we put in the chart."

This difference between the requirements of the chart and what happened on the unit became the focus of a sustained and complex movement of resistance centered on the specific requirements of the chart. Douglass Center charts contained pages labeled "Patient Plan for Treatment" (PPT). Space was provided on these pages for listing the patient's strengths and weaknesses, the goals of treatment, and the unit's plans for reaching the goals; the treatment team was expected to develop a "PPT" in cooperation with the patient shortly after his or her admission. After fifteen days the PPT was to be supplemented by a "data base" consisting of information gathered about the patient's background, social supports, and treatment history. From the staff perspective these expectations of the administration and the state involved the visibility and standardization of the unit's work and were in direct conflict with their need to handle charting efficiently. To understand this conflict we need to consider in more depth what charting is.

One aspect of the chart is its representation of the patient's diagnosis, medication, date of admission, and other information in a way that creates a "case." It constitutes what Foucault calls the dossier, an essential feature of the disciplinary regime of the hospital, school, and prison. The chart is important to the disciplining of individuals because it makes them uniformly visible, organizing them in terms of standardized norms. Thus, it is linked in more than a casual way with diagnosis, for the same process of examining the individual that reveals a diagnosis provides the information in the chart. Examination (whether in school or hospital) . . . "places individuals in a field of surveillance [that] also situates them in a network of writing; it engages them in a whole mass of documents that capture and fix them." (1979:188).[16]

Another aspect of the chart is more subtle than the representation of essentializing features. This is the capturing of the patient's individuality—his words, specific aspects of his life—in such a way that this individuality itself can be considered in a comparative (normalizing) way. As Foucault puts it:

> . . . each individual receives as his status his own individuality . . . [and] is linked by his status to the features, the measurements . . . that characterize him and make him a "case." (1979:192)

This "pinning down of each individual in his particularity" makes the chart into a place where the private world of the patient intersects with a public world of standardized features, where "the individual . . . [is] precisely observed and compared with others" (Dreyfus and Rabinow 1982:156).[17]

One reading of Foucault's analysis of the dossier makes its use into something almost diabolically complete, systematic, and accurate. The subject (prisoner, mental patient, or school child) is completely captured in the dossier, which is systematically used both to describe him and to integrate him into the disciplinary apparatus: "The perfect realization of a panoptical vision would certainly produce the individual as a pure object of information, never a subject in communication . . ." (Lentriccia 1988:82).[18]

But Foucault also suggests other outcomes. On the APU, despite highly systematized rules governing the writing, transfer, and storage of charts, the chart itself was often incomplete, fragmentary, and contested. The way the chart was used resulted in "slippage" away from the intentions of the "system." On the one hand, the chart could become a focus of interest to the exclusion of attention to the patient's individuality; thus, as in this description of a general hospital, "the chart often became an easier and surer source of information" than the patient, "actually seem[ing] to replace the patient at times" (Mizrahi 1986:99).[19] On the other hand, the chart could be ignored, mocked, or treated as a means of resistance and protest. Under these circumstances it became a covertly ironic commentary on its own pretension to transparently represent what staff called the "reality" of the unit.

The PPT, with its clear goals and schedules for treatment, was intended to protect patients by requiring that the staff take them into account in making plans for them. One consequence of the "warehousing" of patients in the past was that their time in the hospital had no end; in the stasis fostered by the old institutions there had often been no goal for treatment. The PPT was designed to document in plain language the reason the patient was in the hospital and what needed to happen so that he could leave. Though the PPT had originated at the state level as part of the movement toward deinstitutionalization, it was perceived by many APU staff to come from the hospital administration.

As a consequence, this meant that it came from "nowhere," from the invisible "they" who made up bureaucratic regulations.

Adding the PPT to the chart was part of a movement in medicine toward the institution of "problem-oriented records" that would record, not just symptoms and diagnoses, but the way these were related to the patient's life as a whole. The problem-oriented record enabled "the experienced physician [to] come to know a patient's life, [to] locate facts derived from the history, physical examination and laboratory tests in the dynamic space in which the patient lives, and thereby convert data into information" (Arney and Bergen 1984:86). The physician is expected to take the total situation of the patient into consideration and to act, as Harrison's *Principles and Practice of Modern Medicine* puts it, as the patient's "guide through an illness" (Arney and Bergen 1984:87).[20] The PPT was a type of problem-oriented record in which the documentation of the psychological and social situation of the patient—his weaknesses, goals, outside support—was a shared task, a matter of agreement between staff and patient.

During much of my stay, the PPT was taken quite lightly, serving mostly as a symbol of how the unit's quick turnover made it different from the other places for which the form was designed. Here's a typical discussion:

■ Sam is telling new students how to fill out the PPT. He says of the section entitled "strengths": "Sometimes we have to struggle to come up with any strengths!" Then he comes to "psychotherapy." Robert makes a noise.

SAM: Don't choke!

ROBERT: Short term.

SAM: You put "Meetings three times a week with X." Now, "activity therapy."

RESIDENT: Pacing.

ROBERT: Bugging the nurses.

ROBERT goes on to say: It took fifteen months to design this thing and it should take three seconds to do. It does help organize things but don't get overwhelmed by how important it is.

SAM: The data base is a big incentive for getting the patient out before fifteen days.

ROBERT: It works pretty well down here; very few data bases ever get written.

Thus the PPT could be used to highlight the particular circumstances of the unit; "organizing things" was good, but it was made clear that the actuality of the unit did not match the form. Because patients' stays were so short, many of the goals suggested by the PPT were unrealistic, and because the unit was so sparse, much of what it took for granted (therapy) was absent.

SAM [to a new student to whom he is explaining the PPT]: As you will discover, "routine ward activities" are "nothing." But put it down.

■   A resident had put "group therapy" in a PPT:

SAM: Well, I suppose "group therapy" might be said to occur, though not really.

RESIDENT: How about milieu therapy?

SEVERAL VOICES: Yeah, twenty-four hours a day!

Because the PPT imposed a time limit (both in terms of how soon it was to be written and in terms of the "data base" required after fifteen days) it became an additional item to consider in planning disposition; it added its interval to the many others demanding attention.

■   A PPT is due.

SAM: Just date it back to whenever it was supposed to be.

RESIDENT: We've got to get him out before Thursday. He's not worth a data base!

It was this remark that prompted Sam's comment at the beginning of this section on "backing the trailer." The administration looked for a particular result with its rules, rules based on assumptions about accountability, therapy, and "information"; these rules were recognized but not considered viable on the APU. The PPT, like the trailer, went in unexpected directions; something intended to benefit patients had the unintended consequence of making them less rather than more cared for. Staff mocked the idea that "forms" could create them as responsible; as Sam said one day when an inspection was coming up, "Everyone look humane!"

Toward the end of Sam's tenure on the unit the administration, facing this inspection, tightened up the emphasis on the PPT. They discovered that the APU was not doing PPT interviews but simply filling out the form cursorily in the patient's absence. The administration demanded that the PPT be done with the patient as intended. Sam tried this; it took forty minutes for the interview and twenty minutes for the writing of the PPT. The PPT was problematic because the unit's rapid turnover involved an emphasis on discharge-planning which started at the moment of admission and usually bypassed many of its categories; since patients were on the unit such a short time, the long admissions interviews required were impractical.

Faced with the administration's insistence, the staff tried to find a compromise. They decided to call staffing the "PPT meeting" but fill out the PPT when the patient was admitted, with the nurse, resident, and perhaps social worker present. Sam said about this decision:

> *There was a lot of dissension and disgruntlement. How can we do this? People were ambivalent. Barbara Wilson wanted to do it properly. The residents were angry about the focus on documents rather than the patient. We're trying to find a way to coexist with realities . . . We have to do a kind of PPT that allows us to function and still satisfies the letter of the law.*

One strategy that was discussed was the use of prearranged categories that could be written automatically onto the forms. Lillian said of this:

> *Before we hadn't got to the point of using cheat sheets [but now] let's have cheat sheets. No one knows what goes on in our meetings. The idea is that the man in the street should be able to understand the plan, and to include what the patient wants. It can be simple; we don't have to put down what doesn't apply here. The senior social worker who signed for me while I was gone [on vacation] came up with some wonderful plans, but they were out of touch with clinical reality here. What's the point of going through a whole bunch of stuff if the patient won't do it?*

Lillian decides, in effect, to sabotage the PPT on its own terms. Instead of writing what is in fact unreality dressed up to look like reality, she suggests that "we don't have to put down what doesn't apply here." The cheat sheets would be simple in a way that would, in fact, correspond to the simplicity of the unit and would thus not be cheating at all.

Like many issues on the unit, this one was never resolved once and for all. After the inspection was over, the administration lessened its pressure for PPT meetings, and the staff continued to use a combination of short interviews and cursory, stereotyped formulae to deal with the requirements of the form.

We can see three layers of resistance in the staff's reaction to the PPT. The first reflected the unit's emphasis on efficiency. The PPT was supposed to both individualize and normalize the patient, catching him in a form, a network of writing; yet, because he moved on so fast, he escaped before the ink was dry. The "data base" required "gathering" what was for staff an absurd amount of information; they were looking for the essential information that would get the patient out (is he a veteran?) not for "strengths" (someone once suggested "strong teeth" for a patient who appeared to have no strengths) that might take months or years of work to develop. Thus staff rejected the vision of guidance that lay behind the problem-oriented record and resisted as mere writing the capturing of the patient's individuality that it entailed. By shortening the required interview, making out the form in the absence of the patient, and stereotyping their descriptions of the patient, they streamlined their approach to the requirement and subverted its intention.

The second layer of resistance was not about the patient. From the staff point of view, the PPT was an exposure of *them*; behind its emphasis on "goals" for the patient's treatment was another agenda: it made their work more visible.[21] It was a requirement that they be "good," that they make "wonderful plans" that would provide group therapy and forty-minute interviews for each patient, and it was a requirement that they document this goodness, showing, in Ben's words, that their "best intentions had been applied toward the patient." Ben gave the state planners the benefit of the doubt, noting that the PPT was supposed to prevent the abuse of patients. He said:

> The intention isn't wrong, it wasn't designed to put an additional burden on anyone. It [just] doesn't accomplish its intention. Yet not to have it would involve such basic trust, and this system is not set up for basic trust.

The system was "not set up for basic trust" in a very fundamental way; patient's lives could be exposed in the chart, the chart could reveal the extent to which the staff were doing their work "properly," and the administration, in its turn, could have its control over the staff revealed (though charts) to state inspectors. Thus, a "principle of compulsory visibility" (Foucault 1979:187) pervaded the institution and made the "dynamic space" of the work lives of the staff available through their charting of the lives of their patients. Staff subverted this by making the form into a perverse teaching device and by using cheat sheets that systematized their role, thus converting the writing itself into a covert commentary on their situation.

Finally, the PPT (and the chart in general) failed to accommodate the element of surprise that was central to the emergent problems the APU encountered. Staff felt that they did things with and about patients that came from an intuitive sense of what was needed and that could not, by their very nature, be written down or explained. Ben gave some examples of situations that required actions of the kind that could not be put into a chart.

> *Last week I made rounds and a student said "Why were you confrontive [toward a particular patient]? Were you doing an 'adult-child' role?" I said, yeah, but really it wasn't. I did what* worked. *They [patients] are dependent, and I responded to that reality.*

> *Two weeks ago I threw [a patient] out [he wouldn't talk to us, and had been in and out for months]. [The outpatient director] was there and he was really upset, worried that this was going to be one of those things, that the administration will call up . . . It was the right thing to do, but the question is, why did you do it? It doesn't fit into the well-intentioned perspective. I can explain it but I can't justify it. [The outpatient director] said, "Yes, it was the right thing to do, but I can't believe you did it!"*

Sam, Ben, and Lillian all speak in these passages of the "reality" of the unit, of what was real but not good, spoken but not written, elusive rather than captured. The unit could be "explained," as Ben was explaining it to me, but it could not be "justified," turned into the kind of knowledge expected by the "well-intentioned perspective" and embodied in the chart.

SIX

Like Migrating Birds

I

We're mandated to do impossible things.

—SAM WISHINSKI

Over one-fourth of the patients who were admitted to the APU were returning to the unit. Some came back so many times that the staff compared them to migrating birds homing in on a favorite tree. Although the staff could produce an empty bed by moving a patient on, eventually that bed was likely to be filled again by the same patient. These repeating patients had a significant effect on the way the unit's staff felt about their work; by returning again and again they made visible, often in very idiosyncratic ways, the problematic nature of the emergency service the APU offered.

A resident drew a picture of a patient leaving the Douglass Center and following a circular path through the various dispositions (jail, home) and back "down" via the court, the police, or "family limits exceeded," returning to "the womb of Mother Douglass." The hospital is pictured as providing "TLC" and "vitamins" (the initials stand for the antipsychotic drugs "Mellaril," "Stelazine," etc.) and money from the Department of Social Services. The hospital is the "womb" that does for the patient what the outside world won't do.

This drawing conveys some of the ironies the staff experienced in relation to the return of patients. We saw that the unit was originally conceived as a crash pad, where patients could receive just what was needed to get them back to independent functioning; it was hoped that chronicity and institutionalization could be avoided by treating them quickly. When Ben talked about the unit as a hotel and Walter drew it

117

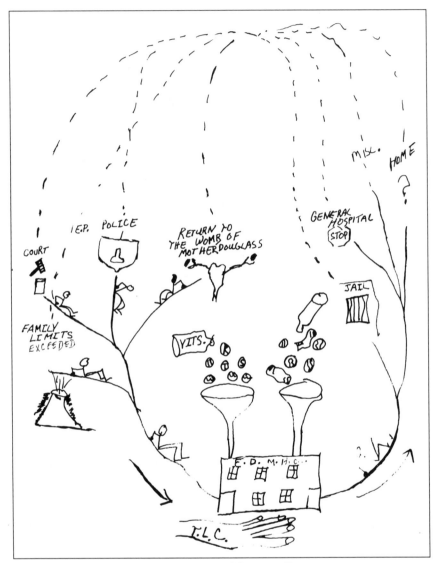

RETURN TO THE WOMB OF MOTHER DOUGLASS

as a funnel they were in alignment with this view of the unit's function. But patients often appeared to resist this definition of the unit as an "oasis" in the "community." The staff said that repeating patients treated the unit as home and came back to it as if it were a "buoy to swim to" in a sea of diminishing resources. In the resident's drawing, the patient's return is depicted as an easy downhill slide toward the care offered by mother hospital.

The staff of the APU were ambivalent and inconsistent in their feelings about returning patients. Sometimes they insisted on the unit's definition as an emergency facility and angrily tried to discourage patients from returning. At other times they resisted the emergency definition, redefining their task to include the periodic nurture of patients who seemed to have developed an emotional attachment to the unit. This redefinition allowed certain patients, like Judge, to contribute a richness of imagery and a continuity of experience that the unit would otherwise have lacked. It did not, however, solve the larger problem, which was that some patients could not be "placed" no matter how great the effort.

Lillian spoke of this dilemma when she complained about a resident who was "doing too much" for patients, trying too hard to make them well once and for all. "You burn yourself out with unrealistic goals," she said. "It can be very cruel when you've got to deal with the real world." She implied that the "real world" was cruel both to the patient, who was unlikely to turn out as the resident hoped, and to the resident, who had to accept his own impotence in the face of patients' repeated failure to meet his goals.

This cruel real world had several interconnected and problematic aspects. The return of patients did not follow an obvious pattern that might have provided an explanation or strategies of prevention. Patients could not be classified as acute cases who were not dependent on institutions and chronic cases who were; from the staff perspective it seemed that almost any patient might return and it was clear that many who did not had simply turned to other facilities. At one point Sam and Ben became intrigued by descriptions in the psychiatric literature of the "young adult chronic patient" who is neither sick enough for long-term hospitalization nor well enough to remain independent (Bachrach 1976). They were confronted by the idea that outside experts had named at least part of what they experienced. But this kind of comfort was fleeting, good mainly as something that residents and medical students could hold on to. The unit's patients were so diverse, the causes of their return so varied, and (often) the conditions of their lives so extreme that theories seemed to have little to offer in the way of concrete suggestions. Patients returned because they stopped taking medication, because they became psychotic or suicidal, because they couldn't find work, because their families would not have them, because they were homeless. The same patient might return, at different times, for any or all of these reasons.

The return of patients brought into constant awareness the inability or refusal of families, other institutions, community care facilities, or homeless shelters to take care of people who were clearly in need. It often seemed to the staff that, as in the case of Judge, the game of "hot shit" ended at the doorway of the APU. Because repeating patients were well known to the staff as individuals, the extent to which their needs were not met by the available resources became very clear. Patients insistently raised the issue Estroff has described as "needs exceeding resources."

> *The American cultural ideal is that adults should have more resources than needs, more money in the bank than is spent . . . Most adult persons whose functioning is restricted . . . break this fundamental rule. Their material, functional, and often social, emotional needs are both exceptional and usually exceed their capacity to provide for them. (1988:20)*

The staff often experienced the "exceptional" needs of patients as beyond any imaginable resource, overwhelming in their intensity and complexity.[1] Paradoxically, in this context the state hospital, which the staff perceived as a permanent placement, took on a kind of glamor. It was the one place that appeared willing to encompass the patient's whole life without expecting him to (partly or eventually) take care of himself.

Patients who returned frequently appeared to identify with their illness and with the hospital, frustrating the efforts of the staff to wean them from "Mother Douglass." The staff wondered whether patients could (or should) be persuaded to modulate their "sick" identity in order to function outside of the hospital, or whether they had to be accepted as they seemed to define themselves. The question was a difficult one. Patients had to be persuaded (or alternatively had to persuade the staff) of their sickness in order to get into the APU; in order to stay out, they had to be convinced that they were well, or at least well enough. When a patient's identity seemed to have become inextricably linked to his diagnosis or when a patient oscillated between a "sick" and a "not sick" identity, the staff felt that their efforts toward discharge were thwarted by the patient's attachment to the hospital.

One medical student followed a patient who left the APU, first for a ward upstairs and later to return to his family. The patient said that he had come to the hospital (voluntarily) because "everyone was rejecting him for speaking his truth" and that he had stopped taking his medication in order to regain "control of his life and his mind." The student expressed frustration that the patient appeared to be "entrenched in his delusion" and was doubtful that the patient wanted to "come down" from his illness.[2] Just before the patient left the hospital the student wrote that "the patient continues to elicit feelings of frustration and anger in me at his seeming unwillingness (inability?) to deal more effectively with his condition." The patient tried to assert an identity separate from his illness ("speaking my truth") and separate from the medication.

Yet the student perceived this identity as a product of illness ("delusional") and was uncertain about whether the patient wanted to change. The student expresses the dilemma in his parenthetical comment about "inability": can't he or won't he? This is the issue central to what Estroff calls the "I am" illnesses, in which there is "a fusion of identity with diagnosis" and "a constriction of social roles and identities to a core of patienthood and disablement" (1988:6). The student shows by his choice of words—"entrenched," "unwillingness/inability," "deal effectively"— that he perceived the patient to be clinging stubbornly to a constricted identity, an identity that the patient, on the other hand, seemed to experience as comforting. In situations like these, the APU staff found that their emphasis on discharge was in conflict with patients' determination to be cared for in ways that confirmed familiar conceptions of self.

Returning patients often seemed to like the unit, at least for a short time. In speaking of these patients the staff developed a metaphor of the unit as home, a warm, familial, almost cozy place, better than anything else available. This image contrasted with the emphasis on barrenness and unattractiveness that was important in many other contexts; if some patients liked the unit so much, it had to be re-imagined in that light. We will see in this chapter that this re-imagining could be difficult and problematic. For under what conditions might such a place seem homelike? Only a stark realization of patients' situations outside the unit could bring sense to this image, yet the staff also had reasons to avoid or minimize such a realization. This ambivalence is described at the end of this chapter in the context of a conflict over the discharge of patients to homeless shelters. In the accounts of the two returning patients that follow, we can see how each patient brought about a confrontation with the question of how the unit could be a home.

II

CHRIS FISCHER

Here we put on a bandaid and send them out.

—WALTER BOYD

The contradictions of patching have no simple resolution.

—HOWARD WAITZKIN (1983:230)

Chris Fischer was a young man from one of the city's working-class neighborhoods. For a while he came into the unit at extraordinarily short intervals, sometimes returning within a couple of days. He had been in and out of institutions all of his life. He was a multiple substance abuser; after overdosing on drugs or alcohol he would become violent, cut his wrists in the police car on the way to jail, and end up in the hospital. He had been arrested thirty or forty times in his short life, usually escaping a court appearance because of his psychotic and self-destructive behavior. He also had bizarre seizures, unresponsive to medication, that the APU staff suspected had evolved as a method of getting into the hospital.

Each time Fischer was admitted he appeared to be extremely sick; he was disoriented, agitated, and sometimes mute. But within two or three days he would begin to act quite normally, so that it was impossible to keep him. And, as Sam said disgustedly, "It's almost arbitrary when he's discharged, he's back in a few days anyway." Thus he represented in an especially acute form the dilemma created by the fact that a patient could only be held in the hospital as long as he was very sick. Many on the unit felt that Fischer had learned how to be "very sick" to escape the law; his chart noted numerous instances of his "slashing his wrists when threatened with return to jail." Sam described him in staffing shortly after one of his admissions:

> He moves constantly from one spot in the system to another. Each part is convinced that they've discharged and deinstitutionalized this guy. Last year I asked him to have people call me; I was getting calls from all over the city—emergency rooms, ICUs for drug overdose . . . He simply does not exist outside the hospital. Last time I bet him that he could not stay out a week and he was back next day. I was prepared to pay him for days out of hospital!

Fischer came into the meeting to be interviewed. He was still in his "sick" phase and was disheveled, sleepy and incoherent.

SAM: Do you know where we are? Have we ever met?

FISCHER: No, I don't think so.

SAM: Follow my finger [a neurological test]. What were you taking, were you sniffing anything? Drinking? PCP? Have you been hurt?

FISCHER [with effort, slurring his words]: I ain't in your world. I'm in another world, a world of death.

But a few days later Fischer was in his "recovery" phase. The staff had been discussing the possibility of long-term care, but feared he would not be accepted because he would seem too "together."

RESIDENT [to Sam]: Fischer wants to see you.

SAM: He wants to manipulate me.

RESIDENT: I think he genuinely likes you.

[Fischer comes in. He is alert, coherent, and personable. He says he's worried about long-term hospitalization because his relatives won't come to see him. Sam points out that they don't come to see him anyway. Fischer says he wants to get out so he can collect his check.]

SAM: What would you use the money for?

FISCHER: Clothes, food.

SAM: I believe you when you make plans here but somehow when you get out on the street it doesn't work out. That's why we're thinking of long-term hospitalization. We'd be pretty stupid not to learn from experience.

FISCHER: I can straighten out myself as long as I stay away from those people and drugs.

SAM: Don't you see how repetitious this is? We've had this conversation before.

FISCHER: I know it, doctor, but I was OK for five months, going to the outpatient clinic.

[Sam points out that it was only two months. They argue about this and Fischer leaves in a huff. Sam resolves to find a long-term placement and assigns to a social work student the task of charting Fischer's history.]

A few days later Lillian found out that Fischer could not be kept in a long-term facility because he was too "well." In the meantime, Sam told me that:

> Bea Radnor suggested another approach—discharge him and tell him if he's in trouble or sick just to come back. We will become a chronic care unit for him—in and out. We'll do brief workups for him and discharge him as soon as he's relatively stable. He would be a chronic patient here. He's about eighteen months old emotionally, has not taken over his self-care, and we are his mother. He hurts himself so he can get cared for, and we have the same reservations about letting him go as for an eighteen-month-old.

Sam didn't accept this idea easily:

> Part of my rage at Chris is that I really do believe that he could be helped. I decided I'm not going to admit him here again, I'm just too angry. I went

*back to Bea and told her my fantasy that [the next time] I would grab him,
drag him across the floor, and fling him into the seclusion room. I knew she
would say, well, I guess you better not readmit him . . . I can send him upstairs.*

Nevertheless, the idea that the unit could be "home" for Chris had a certain appeal. The rest of the staff were willing to consider it. They teased
Sam about his "son, Chris." They thought that at least knowing where
"home" was could be considered a kind of asset in a patient. Lillian saw
a no-fault implication that was the opposite of Sam's offer to pay Chris
to stay well:

*In this capitalist society it's a pyramid, a whole lot are at the bottom. And a
certain percent never get well. But they know where home base is, where to
get nurtured.*

Lillian presented the idea to Fischer.

*He said the other day, "You're getting pretty full, Lillian, throw me out of
here." I said, "Oh no, we're gonna keep you indefinitely. This is home." He
scoffed a little but seemed pretty comfortable with it.*

Fischer inspired three alternating and contradictory impulses on the
part of the staff. The first was rage. He was a "despised repeater," "disgusting" in his ability to manipulate the staff. He was able to move freely
(it seemed to them) into and out of his "world of death," almost mocking
their obligation to help him. They felt that he held a certain power over
them: he knew both how to get in and how to get out of the unit, and
he seemed to deliberately dangle before them the possibility that he
could be helped. Sam, in addition to expressing the outrage Chris
evoked ("he's trying to manipulate me"), tried a countermove, making
his own symptom—"I'm just too angry"—a reason for refusing to admit
him.

The second reaction was an attempt to redefine Chris's relationship
to the unit. Instead of being willing to pay him to stay out the staff could
experiment with accepting him as he was. The unit would become a kind
of intermittent "chronic" placement, a substitute for the state hospital
and a place where he could return freely whenever he liked. The staff
would forego time-consuming admissions interviews and simply let him
back in without fuss. This idea, which came from the inpatient director
in response to Sam's expression of frustration, was immediately re-
phrased on the unit in terms of fatherhood ("your son, Chris"), mother-
hood ("we are his mother"), and home ("this is home"). Perhaps Chris
was really an aggravating eighteen-month-old; seen in this light, his

return did not represent a failure on the part of the staff, but instead suggested that they were engaged in an appropriate kind of mothering. And from this perspective their intense ambivalence—their reluctance to let him out to hurt himself again, and their rage at his return—could be seen as the consequence of a perverse but comprehensible family dynamic.

The staff also found a third response to Chris. The social work student complied with Sam's suggestion and spent weeks developing an elaborate chart, several feet long and drawn with colored pencil, that displayed on a time-line Chris's institutional history. He had been in dozens of psychiatric and medical facilities all over the city and had never been out of the hospital more than a couple of months in his life. This chart became for a while a kind of emblem on the unit. The staff showed it to visitors, and Sam used it for a lecture he gave to a class of first-year medical students.

Chris's chart had a double aspect. It can be understood in part as an attempt by the staff to normalize him by making visible his idiosyncratic relationship to the medical system and by presenting him as an extreme, but knowable, "case." During the time that Fischer was coming to the unit, Sam and Ben were interested in the possibility that returning patients might have predictable intervals between hospitalizations; perhaps the length of time a patient could stay out was part of his identity as a patient, something that the staff could learn to prepare for. Though little progress was made in determining whether specific intervals really existed for most returning patients, Fischer's case seemed to both support and mock the idea of looking for them. He came back so often that knowing his interval seemed of pressing interest, yet his hospitalizations were so close together as to leave almost no interval to be studied.

Although the creation of Fischer's chart can be seen as a normalizing gesture, it can also be understood as a way to represent the hopelessness of the way Fischer's case was being handled, not only by the APU but by the entire "system" through which he drifted. By revealing rather than concealing Fischer's movements, the staff produced a subversive document that contradicted the real chart Fischer already had. By putting his true history on a time-line, they made visible the "impossible" situation that lay behind the admissions and discharges in his official chart and the impossibility of their task. This was the thrust of Sam's lecture to the medical students, in which he presented Judge and Fischer as examples of the kinds of cases he had not been prepared for by his medical training.

After the staff proposed to Fischer that the unit was home he stayed away for over a year. Perhaps he somehow sensed that he was being defined or pinned down and slipped off to less self-conscious facilities. Soon after he stopped coming to the unit another patient, Keith Holmes, caused the staff to take up again the theme of home and mother Douglass.

KEITH HOLMES

Once in a while you seem to make a little more dent than usual in someone; you're not going to cure them, but a little dent.

—DUANE POWERS

There is only room for one person in a psychosis.

—JOHN SANFORD (1977:83)

Keith Holmes was in his middle twenties and came from an inner-city neighborhood near the hospital. Tall and pleasant-looking when I met him, he had, according to Sam, presented a different picture a couple of years before. Then already a veteran of many hospitalizations, Keith looked very "dangerous." He had a "blaze in his eyes" and was "stalking around the ward looking weird and hostile." Sam said:

My first year here I wasn't desensitized to that kind of fear. I wanted him off the ward quickly and got him upstairs right away. By the third year I wasn't fearful of anyone. I can't remember when he became my pet. Maybe finally upstairs didn't want him . . . There was a controversy between us and Day Treatment; they said he was transferred too soon . . . That was the beginning of his becoming our exclusive property. He was basically a chronic patient who could use interminable hospitalization . . . He ceased to be frightening; like a big frightening dog, he sniffs your hand and once he sniffs there's communication . . .

I first met Holmes in November. He had been discharged two weeks before from a ward upstairs where he had been an inpatient since August. They had sent him to Day Treatment (an outpatient program in the hospital), which he had attended only sporadically. His complaint upon admission to the APU was that he heard demons talking to him and couldn't sleep.

Sam suggested that I become a "pseudo case manager" for Keith. This meant that I would follow up on him much as a medical student would, finding out what medicine had worked in the past and exploring options for discharge.[3] This experience brought me into a different relationship to the work of the unit than I had had before; Keith treated me as a member of the staff and I felt emotionally involved with the out-

come of his care. Like Sam, I began full of optimism about him and
ended in despair. In this account I have retained passages in which I
refer to interactions with Keith in terms of "we" and "us," reflecting my
alignment with the staff.[4]

I went to see Holmes's therapist at Day Treatment. He said that
Holmes had never been able to live on his own. He had an apartment
but his mother (the therapist described her as "inconsistent") lived
nearby. Holmes's religious preoccupations were "constant." But the
therapist said that even when he was hearing voices and knew he needed
help, "we can't get him in here." He wondered whether long-term care
at the state hospital would be "less painful to him."

Holmes was a familiar figure on the APU. In a staffing meeting
there was talk about how Holmes had gone home from the hospital with
a girlfriend acquired on the ward and how his claim that demons were
after him for adultery had some substance. Though, as Walter said sar-
castically, "He doesn't let that stand in the way of what he does!" There
was general agreement that "Holmes is *always* like this, in or out of the
hospital."

[Sam woke Holmes from a nap and interviewed him.]

SAM: Day Treatment told us you *sinned*. How?

KEITH: Not attending?

SAM: Right. What penance would wipe it out?

KEITH: Attendance, *good* attendance.

SAM: What other penance?

KEITH: Justifying it to myself, right?

SAM: And God and the Bible? I think you should partake of the sacrament of Prolixin. I could get dressed up for that.

KEITH: You already are.

SAM: I mean I could wear a collar.

KEITH: What's a sacrament?

SAM: Something holy.

KEITH: I'm still asleep; this is like a dream.

SAM: It is a dream.

KEITH: I don't think I have to stay long. I can find a better place to live
and leave.

SAM: You mean you don't think you should live in suffering?

KEITH: Nobody should do that.

SAM: Would it help to live by yourself like a hermit?

KEITH: No, I need a better situation, I need to live on my own for real, instead of depending on my family. My mother wants me to be her little boy, she puts me together with my brothers and sisters. I need to stay away from them.

SAM: You want to get a place to live? Will your demons allow it?

KEITH: I got so much sleep, I can't hear them now.

[Sam pretends that *he* hears them. Keith says that his mother doesn't feed him enough on the money he gives her. Then Keith hears the voices, smiles broadly, and says, "They're external!"

SAM [Imitating "voices"]: Don't say that, about your mother!

KEITH: I didn't hear that!

SAM: She didn't feed you.

KEITH: But it's my responsibility, isn't it?

SAM: Well, you gave her the money.

[Sam asks Holmes how he would feel about a boarding house, and Holmes expresses interest.]

KEITH: Since you're helping me, I'll help myself and look for a room.

This conversation introduced a theme that persisted throughout our interactions with Holmes: his relationship to an inconsistent mother and his desire to be both dependent and independent. This conversation also has a whacky, unlikely tone that continued to characterize Sam's interactions with Holmes. One reason was that Holmes, despite his delusions, was more coherent than most APU patients. He let us in on his thoughts and inspired what the staff called "rescue fantasies"; at times he was so self-aware that we couldn't help imagining him well. Sam was also intrigued with the idea of taking an "inside" position on Holmes's delusions; Holmes was alert to this and responded by playing the part of "rationality." A wonderful expression of whimsical complicity would come over his face when he realized that Sam wasn't trying to talk him out of his experiences.

Sam decided to give Holmes his Prolixin—a shot of antipsychotic medication which lasts about two weeks—in a sort of mock "ritual," tying it into Holmes's religiously oriented delusions.[5]

■   Sam asks Sally for help administering the "sacrament" to Holmes and describes it to her with much joking. She says "He (Holmes) is not crazy, he's a
lazy bum who doesn't want to get off his ass and do anything. And Samuel,
you're not going to do this craziness!" Sam says "That's the point, to act crazier
than he does." Sally immediately grasps the idea, and says, "OK, if you think it
will help." We take Holmes into Duane's office. Sam says: "You've sinned." "No,"
says Holmes. "I need to become an atheist and get myself together." "And the
Prolixin?" "I know the Prolixin helps get enough air to a damaged part of my
brain." Sam says, "This is holy, getting yourself together is also a holy thing."
Holmes is smiling with a look that says "I'm not *this* crazy!" Then he says, pointing to the medicine, "Is this going to make me into a robot again?" "Are you
always?" "Yeah." "And when you don't take it?" "I can't sleep." "How about halfway in between?" Sam tells Sally to give 1½ ccs instead of 2. "This will not make
you into a robot and it will let you sleep" he says to Holmes. "And will you come
to Day Treatment?" It turns out that Holmes doesn't like Day Treatment. Sam
suggests that he negotiate, "on an honest basis" what he wants to do. Sally gives
the shot while Sam, putting on his beret and shawl, plays the accordion. Holmes
laughs and tries to interrupt. "If I feel the pain, what do I do?" he asks. "Come
for help."

The social workers arranged for Holmes to go to a boarding home
for ex-patients. According to Lillian the place had "a home atmosphere."
We talked to Keith before he left. He said that he didn't want to go to
an outpatient clinic; he wanted to come back and see us. Sam said that
he could, "on an informal basis," and set up an appointment with him.
    A week or so later Holmes showed up for his appointment, an hour
early, neatly dressed and looking happy. He talked to us, telling us how
he hated his mother and had always come back to the hospital to get
away from her. He was, he said, the "craziest" of her six children. His
mother would tell him she loved and hated him at the same time, that
he was a sinner and could never be forgiven. He talked a lot about being
a *man*, that he had grown into a man anyway, that he wanted to be a
man; he said he wanted "someone to love" to make up for what was done
to him. He told us about his girlfriend from the hospital and her alcoholism and said he felt there was no future in the relationship.
    Sam said, "What you're looking for is some reliable relatives." "Yes,"
said Keith, "The hospital has been the best mother I have had." Sam
said, "We will try to do that for you and we will tell you if we can't."
    In staffing a few days later Sam described how Holmes came in
"dressed like a pimp" four days early for his next appointment. His eyes
were glittering; he looked hypomanic. He said "Oh, is it Thursday? I'll
just sit out in the lobby." Later he went back to Day Treatment, though
he said he didn't want to stay there. Sam said wistfully, "He looked so
put together last week."
    The next day Holmes reappeared. Sam said, "You need an alarm
clock, a watch, a calendar, and a schedule. So you aren't drifting through

the universe. We need to make out a schedule for you." Sam wrote down the dates of his appointments and made a list. He said, "Do you think you're really gonna do this, or are we making it up?" Keith said, "The last time I made one I couldn't follow it, I was back at State Hospital in a week." Sam added to the list: "Things for you *not* to do: do *not* visit your mother." Holmes said, "What I need is some *friends*."

Five days later Holmes was back on the unit. The boarding home had proved too much for him, and he had stopped taking his extra Prolixin; his shot was due. He had bought a watch but hadn't known how to set it and subsequently lost it. Sam said, "Holmes is the way he usually is; in or out, he's the same." Sam and I talked to Holmes, who was bouncy and cheerful.

SAM: You look better than I feel.

KEITH: How do you feel?

SAM: A sense of lassitude; this depression's not *all* your fault, but . . .

KEITH: You don't need to feel bad, but the decision for the boarding house was rash and uninvestigated.

SAM: What can we learn from it?

KEITH: My decision was based on needing more independence and being hurt.

SAM: We're becoming your family now.

KEITH: I know, the reason I came in is someone's after me . . . I have to plan my life so I can function on my own. I came in . . . some of it was fear.

SAM: When you're here you're OK, you're happy. But what happens outside?

KEITH: I do get confused and start depending on other people to make me feel good and if I don't get that my ambition goes down and I have nobody to encourage me so I lose it. [He talks about how he tried to help his girlfriend and couldn't.] Now I know what a psychiatrist feels like when *they* can't help *me*.

SAM: I thought that's what you were talking about.

KEITH: I like you. But I tried to do your job and I can't handle it, I get too emotionally involved with her; I need her to say she loves me. She doesn't.

SAM: The Douglass Center too?

KEITH: It used to [not love him] but now it gives me approval.

SAM: You got refueled, you came here.

KEITH: For the pat on the back. I can leave now.

SAM [to me]: Maybe the problem is us rather than Keith, if we would let him in a couple of nights a week . . .

KEITH: Well, maybe an annual checkup . . . I don't know what I need. But I don't blame you all, and you all don't blame yourselves.

SAM: The problem is we are on scheduled feeding and you are on a demand feeding schedule.

KEITH [laughing]: Like a baby. I got that watch, but I couldn't get it to work.

SAM: We were saying, come join us in this strange grown-up world. The watch was an invitation. Maybe you don't feel like accepting it now.

KEITH: I wanted two kittens, one called "Keithy," that people would love. I'm trying to raise both of them.

SAM: So they could live together?

KEITH: Yeah, it seems a little dangerous—separating them is cruel. I wouldn't want a dog, but kittens, they can be aggressive, passive, dominant, or submissive. I'm really saying something about myself. I know this'll make you angry: you can't train 'em but you have to let 'em be themselves.

SAM: You can't tell them to come at 2 o'clock.

KEITH: At mealtimes they'll come, but you can't tell them to sit down like a dog. But they'll protect you and help you out.

SAM: You and I'll have a secret agreement—tell me when you want to go, and I'll let you go.

KEITH: A couple of days.

SAM: And when you want to come back, you know how to get in, but if you have any trouble . . .

KEITH: I'd like to pay the bill myself . . .

SAM: No, we learn from you . . .

Later Sam said, "We have to go with the flow; he has a different conception of time. We can't get bent out of shape about it. We should be a timeless unit."

Thus a new conception of Keith took shape. Perhaps his inability to maintain himself and his loose sense of time could be integrated into his relationship with the APU, which would accept his "two sides" as he was trying to nurture his two kittens. As Sam put it:

> We redefined *the indications for rehospitalization from his being floridly delusional to his being distressed outside. We said "We're comfortable with your delusions; are you? Your delusions are OK, but if you're uncomfortable and confused, come in." And we redefined our notion of time—"OK, come when you come, we float in space and time just like you."*

Holmes talked to me about how this redefinition affected him.

> *When I'm in here I feel like I have friends. The outside world seems far away. [Does the outside world look better when you're in?] Yeah, maybe if I get around people who mind their own business my schizophrenia can wear out. Schizophrenia is caused when a person wants to adjust and can't; one side accepts and the other doesn't and, bingo, breakdown. It lasts until the person can be in a situation where they don't have to fight and can rest. One side learns to like the other side. Then comes hope and salvation from one side to another . . . It's a little warmer in here; it's cold out there . . . I get confused about money, time, I'm afraid to learn. If I learned I might lose my mother; she always made me learn her way . . . that's what I think the two kittens are for, to learn from, to get back to what I was before I learned to be stupid.*

Keith and Sam thus articulated several ways of seeing his relationship to the unit. The unit could treat him as a child, substituting for his mother by providing "approval," "love," and "reliable relatives." Keith seemed to respond to this, on the one hand, by asserting that he could take care of himself if he could be in a situation where he didn't have to fight and could rest ("my schizophrenia would wear out") and, on the other, by expressing the fear that "if I learned I might lose my mother"; Mother Douglass, like his own mother, might abandon him if he "got back to where I was before I learned to be stupid."[6] The unit could also treat him as a "pet," someone acceptable, cute, perhaps trainable, a "big dog" who "sniffs your hand." Keith identified himself with his pets, the kittens, but made it clear that he wanted to think of them as somehow independent; he pointed out that they "cannot be made to sit down like a dog," almost as though he had heard Sam's remark to me. Just as a baby could not be scheduled, so "you couldn't train" his kittens. The notion that we were "friends" who would have a secret agreement with him seemed more comfortable; perhaps he could stay out of the "grown-up world" by relating to a "timeless" APU, sharing with us the understanding that "it's a little warmer in here."

Keith's discharge after the discussion of the kittens lasted until Christmas; I was away when he returned. Sam reported on their conversation:

> Keith said that he had done a terrible thing: he had had sex with a dog during a period of psychosis and that was why he was a sinner. He talked on and on about it. Sam said, "How did the dog enjoy it?" Keith looked amazed. Sam said, "Well, you talk as if it's the worst thing in the world but it doesn't sound like a world class sin; the dog survived." Keith said, "I feel better now"; they went back to the nurses' station and Sam discharged him. Then, Sam says, he gave him an appointment to come back and he looked at the calendar wrong and he gave him an impossible date. "It was like saying, come in at 13 o'clock on January 32. He and I are out of space-time. I'm becoming more and more comfortable with craziness: I sat here with Keith and it didn't seem crazy."

Keith pushed further in his identification with pets, perhaps wondering if anything would shock, and Sam became more explicit in his willingness to align himself with Keith's craziness. The interaction is simultaneously crazy and simple; affirmed, Keith leaves immediately. Sam expresses his abandonment of scheduling by giving Keith the kind of appointment Keith himself might make.

It was becoming apparent that we could talk to Keith in this way—enjoying him, proposing increasingly noninstitutional ways of thinking about him—and he would still be back, unchanged, within a few days or weeks. I was beginning to feel the lassitude of repetition. Of what real help were we to him? Was there any situation that could help him? Duane listened to my discouragement and offered the solution he was learning:

> If no one gets better, then you have to redefine success. Maybe you can keep them out for longer and longer periods. I don't look at him as a failure, this is the best he can do and that's OK.

Other members of the staff, who had seen more of Keith over the years, did not share the initial enthusiasm that Sam and I brought to his case. Sally felt that he was simply trying to avoid a normal working life. Walter and Lillian accepted him as a "beloved repeater." They were, however, more practiced than I at holding several feelings about him at once; for them resolution was to be found simply in the gesture of "letting him come back." Lillian said later:

You and Sam liked Keith; we didn't. He showed us our frustration with the system, how deinstitutionalization didn't work. He was marginal, and once we admitted it we could deal with him and work with him, accept him coming back, patch him up for three days or three weeks, and then take him back [again].

For Walter, Judge was always the measuring stick:

Keith was always a pain. Not like the Judge—he was more ambulatory and socialized, had more insight. But his mother made him a pain; I always ended up talking to his mother. He also had a more lovable side, like a teddy bear. I loved Judge out of pity, but Keith was more cuddly. I kind of miss him now, I don't miss the Judge. He was like Ponce de Leon, searching for true love. About him coming back [freely] I was indifferent, he showed up at inappropriate times. He was very manipulative. He was somebody we weren't gonna get rid of; we learned to make the best of it, like the Judge.

Walter was able to hold several contradictory opinions at once, "making the best" of Keith by allowing him to represent both the "lovable" and the "manipulative" side of the repeating patient.

In January Keith came back and, true to Sam's suggestion that he "knew how to get in," he asked for help in killing himself. The resident who admitted him took this seriously, but Lillian explained that Keith "was always the same." She said simply, "He needs to come in from time to time." In this visit Keith kept to his usual pattern. When I went to visit him in the day room a few hours after his admission he was haggard and incoherent; he said that he'd been hearing the voice of Satan and was depressed. But a few days later he was skipping behind the window, smiling broadly. Somehow I didn't feel like talking to him. The others watching from the nurses' station joked that he was back to his "usual level of functioning—a two on a scale of ten!"

Keith continued to come in and out freely for several more months. As Sam put it:

His tie was strong enough so he would come back, not that he was [getting] well but that the tie was sufficient. He was a "beloved repeater" because of his history with the unit, his being big enough to take care of himself. He knew how to survive, how to come back. He had a quality of playfulness. And he associated us with relief from distress.

Sam felt that "this could have gone on indefinitely." But as he prepared to leave the unit, his interest in Keith waned. In March Keith came in one day when the APU was full and Sam sent him upstairs. Duane was disturbed and saddened. He said, "When Holmes comes in, Sam should kick someone else upstairs so Holmes can be here. It is not good for him to be upstairs, he'll lose his apartment . . ." But the deed was done.

Thus the APU was, after all, an unreliable family, a home that could not be counted on. Keith was on a ward upstairs for several months; finally he was admitted to the long-term unit at State Hospital. Lillian said:

> *[The staff of the ward upstairs] got tired of dealing with him. He is a fail-ure of deinstitutionalization. Some people are better off at State Hospital whether they are young or old. They go out on the grounds, three meals, and they do what they want. You can lolligag out there and you still get your medicine.*

Ben called the approach that Sam instituted with Keith "the city as grounds." At the state hospital, he said, patients were free to roam the grounds, coming back to the wards for meals and bedtime. For patients like Keith the city had become the grounds in which they wandered, coming back to the unit regularly for rest and refueling. "You can go," said Ben, "as far as you can get in a day."

In this experience with Keith the staff gradually worked out in prac-tice this attitude toward the city and its facilities; instead of being angry that he could not stay out, as they had been with Fischer, they began to see his apartment and his mother as stopping-places on the way back to the APU. Keith contributed to this understanding by making it clear that the "warmth" of the APU enabled him to regain his equilibrium and, briefly, to try again. The staff found that they could see themselves as competent, not just for moving patients out, but also for understanding them when they came back. During the latter part of Keith's relationship with the unit Sam reported this conversation with another repeating patient:

> *[The patient] told me about what he called the "via-calm conveyance," de-scribing the Douglass Center as the calm hub of the universe on which a variety of "conveyances" converged. As he elaborated his delusion it corre-sponded to my view; this guy in his rambling flight of ideas described the function of the place. An outside observer might see this as crazy, but he had [an] insight.*

This attitude is quite different from that of the student quoted earlier who was frustrated when his patient "wanted" to stay delusional. Keith was, with other repeating patients, the "teacher" of an inverse competence; patient's delusions and idiosyncracies could form the basis for a different, but valid, understanding of events. Sam at first assumed that when Keith asked for a "mother" he was asking to be socialized into the routinization of a normal life. The "reality-testing" of the Prolixin ritual, the attempt to regularize Keith's sense of time, and the writing down of what needed to be done were all normalizing strategies. But Keith resisted efficiency and asked us to join in his definition of the situation. He was, at least temporarily, party to a "secret agreement" about what the unit was for.

It was characteristic of the unit that the agreement, however contextualized and metaphorically rich, was in fact temporary and contingent. The staff worked out a relationship with Keith as though they "couldn't get rid of him," but actually they did get rid of him. In retrospect, it is hard not to see a certain hallucinatory quality in Sam's conversations with Keith, with their dreamlike play on the metaphor of home.

III

Ben and Sam are basically good, but they are too cynical. There must be some other way to do this work without burning out.

—ANTHONY GIULIANI

For the APU staff the ambiguities surrounding the unit as home had as a corollary the problem of how to think about the outside world. Was the city the equivalent of the benign grounds of the state hospital, a place where patients could probably manage temporarily? Or did the city in fact provide "placements" where patients were subjected to scrutiny, hostility, and extreme conditions?

Some dispositions were unacceptable to patients or to the administration, yet the APU staff regarded them as the only option available. This was the case with the "mission," a place that became the focus of a conflict between the administration and the unit. The mission was the largest facility of its kind in Midway City and was about twenty blocks away from the Douglass Center. It was an old building in a rundown neighborhood, with two large rooms packed full of iron beds, each with a mattress and a single blanket. In the basement was a kitchen and a primitive dining room, where a missionary read scripture before dinner. The mission could take eighty men a night.

We saw in chapter 2 that the staff discharged some patients to the mission if they had nowhere else to go and if there was pressure to get the patient out. This discussion is typical of the way the mission might be considered as an option.

STUDENT: [The patient] is doing well and he can go, but we can't get hold of his relatives, there's no phone. If I can't get hold of his relatives, shall I discharge him to the mission?

SAM: Is he up to that? Where was he before?

STUDENT: He was with his wife but they weren't getting along

LILLIAN: Let him know what he's getting thrown into and maybe he'll come up with somebody.

STUDENT: . . . Now he understands that he has to be followed and take meds.

SAM: Why don't you talk to him about the mission and tell him if things don't work out he can come back. Let him go early in the day tomorrow and he can come back later if things don't work. Unofficially hold a bed. . . . We went through this last year and he said he didn't want to go back to his wife but he lived with her all year.

This use of the mission had both a persuasive and a practical aspect. If the patient had no immediate place with relatives, and he could handle it, the APU staff felt comfortable sending him to the mission until some other place became available. But there was also the likelihood that the patient would be galvanized into action by the possibility of discharge to the mission. Proposing the mission thus provided either a direct or an indirect solution to the disposition problem. It was treated as another unpleasant place linked to the unit by the patient's passage back and forth.

One of the things that made "despised repeaters" "disgusting" to the staff was their "manipulation" in trying to remain in the hospital. Duane reported on one patient:

> This patient says he will kill himself if sent to the mission. He recently left a ward upstairs and stayed at the mission, where he began using heroin again. If he's outside, he has no place to stay but he can get drugs. If he's inside he has a place to stay but no drugs. His adaptive solution is to go back and forth.

Duane tried to work with the patient on his drug addiction, but when, after two weeks, the patient remained resistant, Duane said disgustedly, "This guy's hopeless, I'm sending him to the mission." The mission was part of an "adaptive solution" that the patient appeared unwilling to give up.

An initially sympathetic assessment of a patient could give way to disgust upon further investigation. In this discussion the revelation of the patient's drug addiction and suspicion that his symptoms are deliberate lead the staff to an insistence that the unit not be treated as "home" by a patient who, in their view, "deserved" to go to the mission.

CASE WORKER: There's still no place to send him but a mission.

SOCIAL WORK STUDENT: What does he want to do?

CASE WORKER: Ideally a place to live but he's worried about going out. He doesn't want to go to the mission. He got money from the homeless unit [welfare] but he blew it on cocaine.

ROBERT: He didn't actually blow it, he inhaled it!

SAM: This puts a new light on him; it seemed unfair [to send him out] but it's a consequence of what he did.

SOCIAL WORK STUDENT; He's afraid to go to the mission so he's hearing voices.

RONNIE: I notice that whenever he thinks it might be his turn to be discharged he goes to his room with "hallucinations."

ROBERT: Throw him out.

SAM [to student]: What do you think?

STUDENT: Discharge him; he can stick it out at the mission for the rest of the month.

SAM: Could you provide follow-up, have him come in until next month when he has money [a welfare check] and talk to Walter about his eligibility for a drug program. Let's plan his discharge for tomorrow.

The patient in this discussion hovers in a no-man's land: is he mainly (really) crazy? Is he mostly homeless? Or is he deliberately using the unit to solve a problem caused by his drug addiction? The staff use the option of the mission to avoid what they see as the patient's attempt to define himself as crazy.[7]

Eventually, the mission complained to the Douglass Center about discharged patients who became psychotic and disruptive in their care. Bea Radnor sent a memo to the unit saying that patients were no longer to be discharged to the mission. This "mission memo" angered the APU staff. They felt that she did not understand what they were dealing with. During a discussion in staffing, one of the residents mentioned that when he took this up with Bea, she conceded that the mission might have to be a last resort, but said that any referrals to the mission had to go "through her."

SAM: Well, if you get a patient with nowhere to go and say, "Aw, shucks, I can't keep this patient who's signed a voluntary," you can call Bea Radnor and say, "There's nowhere else for this patient to go." She may hem and haw but . . .

In the end, he implied, she would bow to the reality of the situation: a voluntary patient could not be kept against his will, whether he had an acceptable place to go or not.

The mission memo was like the PPT in making visible the actual practice of the staff; as with the PPT there was disagreement and ambivalence about how much to "hide" from the administration. This discussion in staffing took place after the mission memo had been received; sending a patient to the mission was no longer a simple matter:

LILLIAN: The only option we have to offer [this patient] *is* the mission. Or to get a more suitable situation he'll have to be here a long time.

STUDENT: So just give him that option.

DUANE: You tell him he's got to work on disposition *now*: it's his responsibility to get on the phone.

LILLIAN: I have no patience with this guy; I was hard on him.

DUANE: Tell him he has three options: mission, upstairs, or his friends.

ROBERT: Two options, mission or friends.

LILLIAN: You have to offer him Bea Radnor . . .

ROBERT: But is he in need of psychiatric hospitalization?

DUANE: Less and less.

LILLIAN: Bring it up with Radnor.

DUANE: I listen to what Radnor says.

LILLIAN: Duane has to protect himself.

STUDENT: So I'll give him a deadline of Friday.

DUANE: It's not your job [placement]; he can always use the phone . . .

ROBERT: There's a third option—if he says no and refuses to leave, arrest him for trespassing!

SOCIAL WORKER: So then he'll be here on court order!

These staff members feel that this patient is angling to be sent upstairs; he wants to be in the hospital a "long time," while they want him to take responsibility for finding a place. The mission still serves a purpose, but now Radnor has also been incorporated into the strategy. She will have to let the patient go if he does not need to be hospitalized, but everyone knows that Duane, dependent on her for recommendations and in a position of legal responsibility, would be unwise to ignore the memo altogether.

Thus the mission became, like the chart, another contested, unsettled territory, the site of an uneasy truce between the pragmatic world of the unit and administrative responsibility. Ben explained the relationship between the use of the memo, the issue of visibility, and the problem of returning patients:

> *When we do things here we usually don't get caught. The mission memo comes from being caught. Here you're colluding on practices that are not bad but unapproved. If word gets out they have to be responded to. Anthony and Bea don't come down here. They think they know but they don't—there's a collusion above us not to look, to remain ignorant. But when someone spills the beans—like the mission calls that a psychotic got out—you have to show you're a* good *person . . . Once a mission calls then the catchword is "aftercare," which means a promise that the person won't ever come back. The closer you are to the patient the more you know that's bullshit. This [situation] gets framed up [by the administration] in terms of "aftercare" and leads to questions like "Why are we such bad clinicians? Didn't we learn anything anywhere?" The point is we did but we can't tell anyone about it.*

The staff couldn't tell anyone about the kind of competence they felt in relation to patients like Keith, or about their skill in what they felt were legitimate uses of the mission. The complaint of the mission made visible to the administration the fact that there was no "aftercare," no "promise that the person won't ever come back," whereas on the unit "closeness to the patient" meant that one identified his true, rather than his imaginary, options.

Anthony Giuliani took an entirely different position. For him the "outside" was the state and the danger was that the hospital's situation would be misrepresented. Giuliani felt that the mission provided a spurious placement that gave the Mental Health Department the misleading impression that patients had places to go. Furthermore, he thought of the patients as vulnerable, like children, and of the staff as alarmingly ready to eject them into a hostile environment. He blamed the APU for neglecting aftercare:

> *I believe we should not be too quick to give up finding suitable places for patients in the community. We should keep them here if necessary and keep others out to create an explosion outside [that is, to direct community attention to the lack of places]. The fewer patients we discharge, the fewer we admit. So we can present a tangible argument to the establishment. This argument is diffused by placement. In addition, it is cruel to send patients*

to the mission. Everyone [on the unit] feels OK about it, but they've done nothing for the patients . . . In the missions they have no support. It's revolting to me. If the patient wants to go, that's a different matter. But some patients don't have the capacity to think it through and may not know how damaging it is for them. The APU has the worst record [in the hospital] on patient aftercare continuity—it's not a value for them, they don't feel it's important. They don't feel the way you would about a relative.

For Giuliani the mission, not the patient, was disgusting. He reverses the direction of Keith's conversation with Sam, saying that the staff should treat the patients like "relatives"; for Giuliani this means not only that the patient is dependent but that he may not know what is good for him. Giuliani felt that Ben and Sam were able to send patients to the mission because they kept a cynical distance from them, not because, as Ben believed, they were "close" enough to consider "aftercare continuity" to be "bullshit." Giuliani was also a strategist, however; the back-up of patients "outside" had value for him as a message to those above him that resources were inadequate. Giuliani believed that better psychiatric facilities would result if only the real situation could be made visible.

For the APU staff, on the other hand, the mission remained an option, even if a hidden one. From their perspective the use of the mission reflected the real situation of homeless patients and the real situation of the unit in its dealings with the erratic connection between returning patients and the hospital.

SEVEN

It Is Impossible
To Be Good

I

We speak, glibly, of "institutionalization," without the smallest personal sense of what is involved—how insidious, and universal, is the contraction in all realms (not least the moral realm), and how swiftly it can happen to anyone, oneself.

—OLIVER SACKS (1984:157)

If you think these are people, what an awful life! If you stop thinking of them as objects and think of what it would be to live that life . . .

—DUANE POWERS

A resident made a drawing of the window that separated the nursing station from the patients' hallway. The back of the unit is shown as an aquarium, with patients the fish swimming behind the glass and making requests like "Can I go back to jail?" Next to the door, apparently waiting to be used, is a fishing pole.

The aquarium window was the site of a mutual gaze in which the staff confronted the otherness and difference of the patients. This confrontation did not always yield to the panacea, "Remember, *you* are not the patient." The window seemed to divide the staff from the patients. But patients could "sneak up from behind" in less literal ways than Mr. A, forcing staff to acknowledge the inner landscapes on their own side of the glass.

Whether the staff thought of the patients, in Duane's words, as objects or as people, they found themselves facing uncomfortable questions about themselves. If the patients were seen as people, then their immersion in craziness and poverty pointed to the ways that anyone could come undone. Ben spoke of the "fear of craziness" that made new residents behave in rigid or authoritarian ways. The patients aroused strong emotions of anger or pity and called up responses that were dormant in everyday interactions (cf. Stamm 1987; Stein 1985). On the other hand, if the patients were seen as objects, then the staff had made them so and could not remain within the "well-intentioned perspective." They had to consider that perhaps their position was closer to that of prison or concentration camp guards than healers.

Thus the window could also be a mirror, reflecting the staff to themselves. Their experiences on the unit challenged the everyday assumption that personhood is singular and context-free, as the patients seemed to call up responses that were dormant in ordinary interactions. The patients raised for the staff the possibility that they harbored alternative selves that would not meet with approval outside the unit (cf. Harre 1980; Scheinfeld et al. n.d.).

Ben and Sam were self-conscious in articulating this aspect of their practice; they were influenced by psychoanalysis in their thinking about their own reactions, and they had the most flexibility and authority to behave spontaneously on the unit. For other staff members the issues were more likely to come out in direct expressions of anger and humorous parody. Whether mediated by self-conscious reflection or not, the emotional reactions of the staff to patients whom they considered particularly difficult suggest that these patients called into question fundamental assumptions about the nature of the self. Particularly at issue was the relationship between the self and work. Patients seemed to have abdicated responsibility for themselves, while the staff, asked to take responsibility, found that to do so raised intractable problems of agency.

THE VIP TREATMENT

> . . . *everyone is caught, those who exercise power just as much as those over whom it is exercised.*
>
> —MICHEL FOUCAULT (1980:156)

> *Use your limitations.*
>
> —BEN CALDWELL

One of the first things Sam told me about the unit was that occasionally a patient was placed on "room restriction" (that is, forced to stay in his room), deprived of cigarettes, and given a restricted, 1200-calorie diet with no salt. This treatment was called the "VIP" treatment and was, he told me, one way that the unit responded to patients who "misused" the hospital.

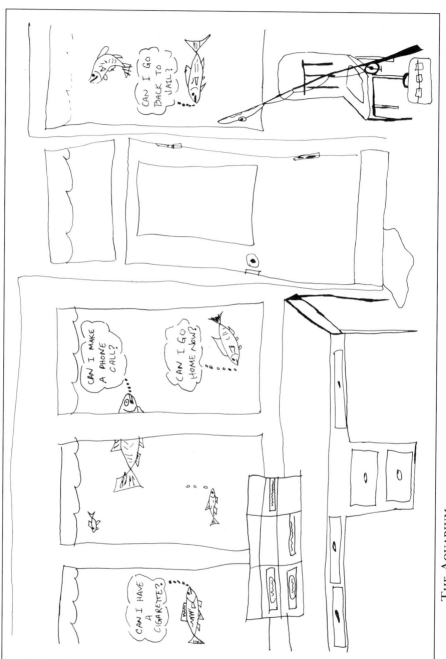

THE AQUARIUM

The VIP treatment was invented by Ben to handle repeating patients with a history of drug or alcohol addiction who were, he felt, using the unit as a place to rest. They manipulated the staff by saying "I'm gonna kill myself if you don't take care of me." The VIP treatment was one of the ways Ben made the place "not a cradle." In the early days of the unit, if anyone questioned him about it, he gave a reason like "history of ulcers."

Sam's image of the unit as a "perverse monastery" originated with his experience with the VIP treatment. When he arrived on the unit he felt that it was a "brutal" idea. But, like Ben, he discovered the frustration of dealing with "despised repeaters." In response, he developed a strategy that not only "tried to convert the VIP to an actual treatment" but produced what he considered his only "cure" during his entire tenure on the unit.

The patient was an alcoholic and not, Sam stressed, psychotic.[1] Sam described his decision to try it:

> I wouldn't do it [the VIP treatment] for a while, I felt very uncomfortable, I felt I was crazy doing it, because it was so very alien to what I had done before. But it was desperation. He had come back a lot, again and again. Also, I spoke to the alcohol counselor and she said, "Oh, he's hopeless, everything has been tried, he's no-account, no good." But he was not psychotic, there was no indication for medicine. I think when there's an indication for medicine I have a hope, I have a magical hope about medicine that they [might] get better. But I couldn't justify giving him anything. Plus, he was so self-pitying and blaming of others and his reason for not working was one which made me particularly angry. He had had a leg injury and it was a very mild injury and he told me that he couldn't work because of his leg. And here I am limping around here and he didn't notice that, it never occurred to him that he should be able to work if I could.

Sam restricted the patient to his room and told him to write in a notebook all the reasons he was sick. For three days the patient wrote "his excuses."

> I told him it was bullshit and to write it again. I would stomp my cane on the floor and tell him it was bullshit and make him write it again. I was really putting pressure and I was enjoying it too. One morning he was crying and saying, "Thank you, thank you." He saw the light. I felt like a Zen master who says, "That's not it, struggle some more."

The patient pulled himself together and left the unit, never to return. He got a job, and when Sam ran into him a year later he expressed great appreciation for his treatment.

A resident who was uncomfortable about the way the unit operated told Anthony Giuliani about the VIP treatment. He went, Sam said disgustedly, "with tears in his eyes and said, 'Do you know what they're doing to the patients down there?'" Giuliani was appalled. He told Ben to put an immediate stop to the treatment. To me he said furiously, "Would you do this to your children? The patients are no different from our children!" Sam said:

> *The resident blew the whistle on me. Everyone liked it until then and he did too [that is, it was practical] but [telling] was his best weapon [to express his overall displeasure with the unit].*

For a time the VIP treatment went into disuse, though it was sometimes mentioned as a possible treatment of last resort. But a year later, there was this discussion in staffing:

■ The resident admitted a patient "for VIP treatment—room restriction, low calorie diet, no salt, and no cigarettes. He's going to write his life story." This was in response to a history of coming in saying he would kill himself, getting in, then changing his mind in a couple of days. He is an alcoholic.

STUDENT: [Patient] is on the VIP treatment.

SAM: Which doesn't exist, but nevertheless . . . Has he sobered up? Talk to him today, check his motivation.

STUDENT: This guy has been to State Hospital more than ten times for alcohol detox; unless he's put somewhere [that is, locked up] he won't attend any abstinence meetings.

SAM: Run it through anyway—tell him we'll ask him again [to write his excuses] next time and the time after that . . .

The VIP treatment persisted despite strong sanction and was spoken of much more frequently than it was used. The idea had an attraction that seemed to go beyond whatever practical use it might have had in isolated cases. Part of the attraction seemed to rest in the notion that the expression of emotion, especially negative emotion, might be beneficial. In some ways the VIP treatment resembled the seclusion of Mr. A. Both patients were confined against their will, and in both cases the staff avoided identification with the patient in order to exert their will over him. In both cases it was hoped that confinement would change the patient, either by revealing his true symptoms or by providing him with an opportunity for insight. But Renee was asked to distance herself, to swallow her pity in the interests of an objective understanding of her patient. Sam, on the other hand, acted on his anger. He allowed the patient to affect him and pointed to the patient's cure as evidence that this was not a mistake.

The VIP treatment also had a meaning that ran somewhat contrary to this confirmation of the usefulness of emotional expression. It resembles the handling of madmen in the early nineteenth century, when patients were, for the first time, expected to exercise restraint upon themselves. The VIP treatment brought the crudest institutional constraints to bear on the patient, but it did so in a context of moral expectation. The disciplines of silence, abstinence, and writing, imposed in an enclosed space, were the means by which the patient was required to remake himself. The possibility that this exaggeration, almost parody, of the unit's everyday offering could work, even once, was another source of its fascination for the staff.

II

. . . the meaning of life for most Americans is to become one's own person, almost to give birth to oneself.

—ROBERT BELLAH (1985:83)

If you've never worked with anyone not motivated to change and then you run into folks with none or so very little (motivation) it can be quite startling.

—ROBERT NAUMANN

The VIP treatment raised a question of responsibility that pervaded many less drastic interactions with patients. Were the patients like children, as Giuliani insisted? Psychotic and severely impaired patients like Judge sometimes behaved like children, and such behavior legitimized their presence on the unit. When Trina said, referring to the Judge, that "we have some really sick people here," she said it proudly. But with many patients the situation was not so clear; they seemed to require one to think of them *both* as choosing their own fate *and* as passive victims of circumstances. Sam portrayed this contradiction in a board game called "Mental Patient" that he invented during his first year on the unit.

The game is described as "exceedingly tedious, repetitive, and demoralizing," but many people "choose to devote decades of their lives to it." The "choices" presented by spinning the wheel suggest that patients do have control over themselves, as in "you avoid alcohol" and "compliant" (with medication). But the game is also a whimsical representation of the double binds created by legal, economic, and medical

Rules: MENTAL PATIENT is an exceedingly tedious and repetitive game, demoralizing to its players. Nonetheless many people choose to devote decades of their lives to it.

The object is to escape from the game. Suicide is not permitted.

The game is equipped with a spinner specially designed by an artist with a right hemispheric lesion.

Spins are indicated by ⬭ blocks

1-3 ↙   4-10 ↘

The numbers along the arrows indicate which path to follow.

The Street

↓

You avoid alcohol → No → Accumulate 10 cirrhosis & 5 organicity points → Go to decompensate

↓

You avoid PCP → No → Accumulate 2 organicity points →

↓

You avoid LSD → No →

↓

DEATH: Congratulations — you have finally succeeded in destroying yourself, to the relief of your family, the state, and best of all yourself. For at last, in your own way, you have succeeded in escaping the game.

THE GAME OF MENTAL PATIENT

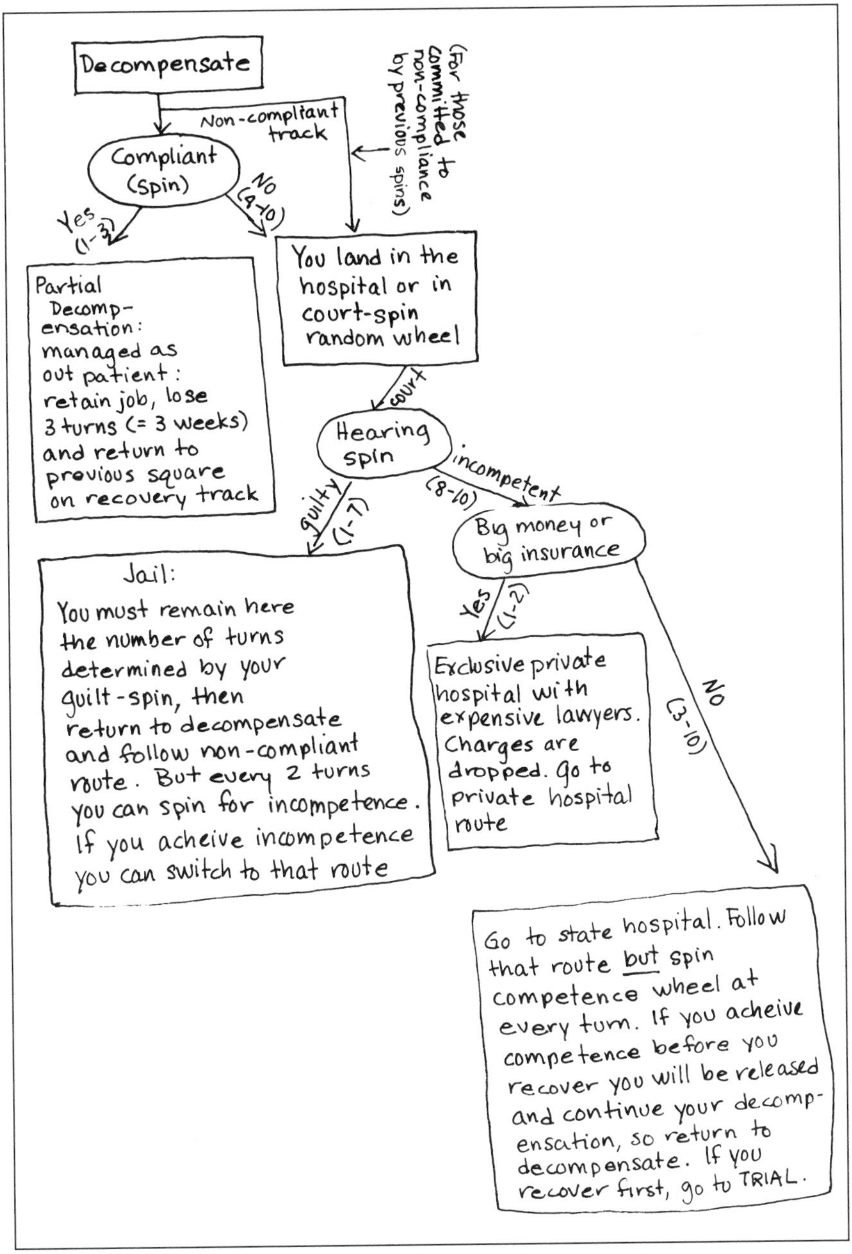
Decompensate
Non-compliant track
(For those committed to non-compliance by previous spins)
Compliant (spin)
Yes (1-3)
No (4-10)
Partial Decompensation: managed as out patient: retain job, lose 3 turns (= 3 weeks) and return to previous square on recovery track
You land in the hospital or in court-spin random wheel
court
Hearing spin
guilty (1-7)
incompetent (8-10)
Big money or big insurance
Yes (1-2)
No (3-10)
Jail: You must remain here the number of turns determined by your guilt-spin, then return to decompensate and follow non-compliant route. But every 2 turns you can spin for incompetence. If you acheive incompetence you can switch to that route
Exclusive private hospital with expensive lawyers. Charges are dropped. Go to private hospital route
Go to state hospital. Follow that route but spin competence wheel at every turn. If you acheive competence before you recover you will be released and continue your decompensation, so return to decompensate. If you recover first, go to TRIAL.

THE GAME OF MENTAL PATIENT (continued)

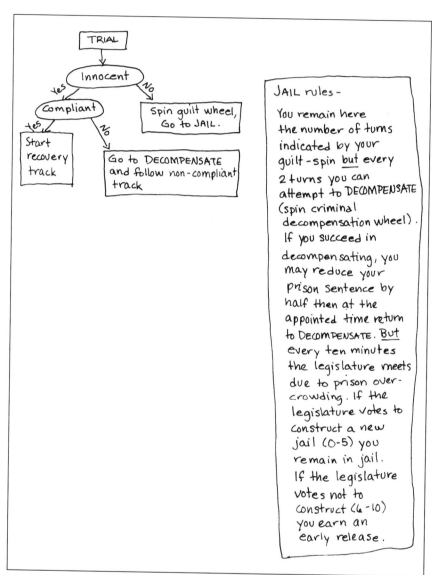

TRIAL

Innocent

Yes ↙   ↘ No

Compliant

yes ↙   ↘ No

Start recovery track

Spin guilt wheel, Go to JAIL.

Go to DECOMPENSATE and follow non-compliant track

JAIL rules—

You remain here the number of turns indicated by your guilt-spin <u>but</u> every 2 turns you can attempt to DECOMPENSATE (spin criminal decompensation wheel). If you succeed in decompensating, you may reduce your prison sentence by half then at the appointed time return to DECOMPENSATE. <u>But</u> every ten minutes the legislature meets due to prison over-crowding. If the legislature votes to construct a new jail (0-5) you remain in jail. If the legislature votes not to construct (6-10) you earn an early release.

THE GAME OF MENTAL PATIENT (continued)

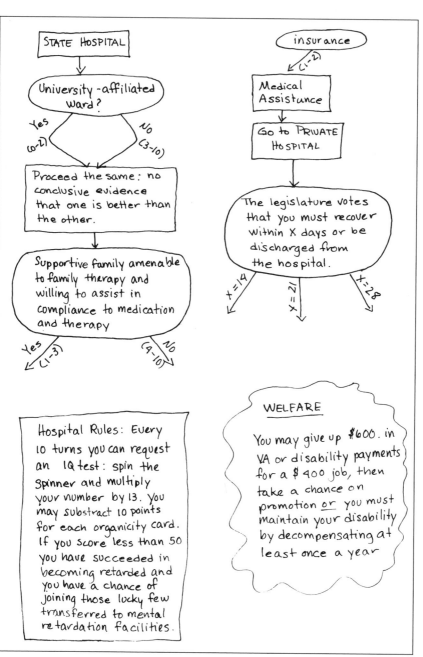

STATE HOSPITAL

University-affiliated ward?

Yes (6-2)   No (3-10)

Proceed the same: no conclusive evidence that one is better than the other.

Supportive family amenable to family therapy and willing to assist in compliance to medication and therapy

Yes (1-3)   No (4-10)

insurance

(1-2)

Medical Assistance

Go to PRIVATE HOSPITAL

The legislature votes that you must recover within X days or be discharged from the hospital.

X=14   X=21   X=28

Hospital Rules: Every 10 turns you can request an IQ test: spin the Spinner and multiply your number by 13. You may substract 10 points for each organicity card. If you score less than 50 you have succeeded in becoming retarded and you have a chance of joining those lucky few transferred to mental retardation facilities.

WELFARE

You may give up $600. in VA or disability payments for a $400 job, then take a chance on promotion or you must maintain your disability by decompensating at least once a year

THE GAME OF MENTAL PATIENT (continued)

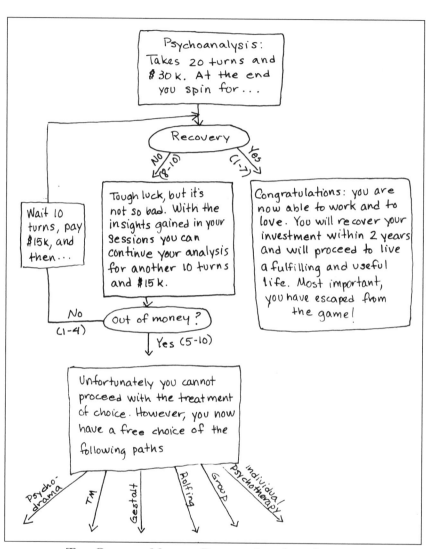

THE GAME OF MENTAL PATIENT (continued)

constraints. You can "take a $440 a month job or maintain your disability by decompensating once a year." You can "succeed in becoming retarded" or "succeed in destroying yourself." The game presents only two routes to "escape" (not counting death)—compliance with medication and psychoanalysis, ironically presented as a circular scramble for money. However, if you get well through psychoanalysis, you "will recover your investment within two years" through your newfound ability to "work and live a useful life."

The game suggested the distance between the cultural ideal of living a useful life and the real lives of the patients. But it also played on the question of choice and on the fact that some patients had developed a perverse redefinition of "success." One APU patient, a wanderer of unknown identity, called himself "Mr. Competencies," mockingly suggesting both his incompetence in the world of work and his proficiency at dealing with the world of institutional care. These patients, who seemed to care for themselves mainly by obtaining care from others, seemed to require, even to demand, "discipline," regimentation, and confrontation.

The confrontation often centered around work. One day in staffing Sam told a story about a man he saw who had cerebral palsy and who was struggling across the street *to go to work*. There were sarcastic comments from every corner of the room: "We should have a video of that and play it two times a day!" One of the residents said, "We could make a background of one of our patients whining, 'What, work? I get a *check!*'" Elaborating a similar theme, Ronnie told me that one day she saw a man in a wheelchair selling newspapers; she had previously seen him begging. When he was begging she had refused to give him money, because "being in a wheelchair doesn't make you an invalid," but she bought a paper from him because "he was doing something" for himself. The occasional patient who was holding down a job aroused open admiration on the unit.

Patients' small gestures of self-reliance, such as making a phone call to the welfare office or reading the newspaper, were often taken by staff to represent the larger issue of autonomy. Lillian was particularly sensitive to these gestures, or more often to their absence, because many patients expected her to act the part of the "take-charge social worker." In the following discussion she takes the lead in expressing intense frustration with the dependency of a patient, articulating the value placed by staff on autonomy and productivity. The patient returned to the unit often and was well known to everyone as a "despised repeater." Renee begins by taking the patient at his word.

RENEE: Thompson still doesn't know where he is; I don't know if he's capable of going out. Sometimes he knows where he is, sometimes he has a machine in his brain.

LILLIAN: Thompson has got on my one black nerve. He is full of shit. We gave him [the number of a group home] the only place he might be appropriate for. Thompson comes in this morning and says "I called her yesterday and I can't remember what she said. Maybe you should call, I've got a memory problem, you do it." I said, "Let me tell you something, you are expecting us to do everything. We'll help you, but *you have to do for yourself.* You might as well leave now if you think we'll do for you." Maybe he should just go to a mission and when he decides to assume some responsibility he can come back. He would probably ask us to breathe for him, *he is disgusting!* [apologetically] I don't usually get so hostile.

DUANE: You don't like him.

LILLIAN: No, I don't.

DUANE: I don't either.

RENEE: He understands and does what will get him what he wants. He'd be very comfortable right here on the unit for eighteen months.

LILLIAN: Give me back the Judge!

RONNIE: He's one of the longest; we've filled this place three times since he came in. There's nothing wrong with his memory. [She mimics him saying "I'm confused."]

DUANE [to another resident]: Your job is to get this piece of shit out of here.

RONNIE: If he wants to act out sexually, let him do it in the community!

DUANE: Let him call the home again and give him two options, that or walking to the mission. We don't have enough staff to help him if he can't help himself.

LILLIAN: We can tell him that but in the end we have to drive him [for legal reasons].

DUANE: Get tough with him.

RONNIE: In two more days you've gotta do a data base.

LILLIAN: Ooh, they're awful. Six pages.

DUANE: You gotta jump on him.

In this discussion the patient's refusal to help himself is the focus of the staff's outrage. They contrast what they feel were the legitimate needs of the Judge with this patient's manipulation; they are forced to do unnecessary work (making calls, driving him, writing up the data base) for someone they feel is capable. They describe the patient as a strategist against whom countermoves must be planned.

The unit did not usually try to foster changes in patients' habits, other than insisting that they take responsibility for moving on. But sometimes the connection between discipline, hospitalization, and self-knowledge was made very clear.

■ King James exposed himself at a local hospital and was readmitted to the unit. The staff came up with a plan to restrict his cigarettes and reward him with them for writing in a journal.

SAM: He can earn his cigarettes.

RENEE: You mean you're gonna make him earn his *own* cigarettes?

LILLIAN: I think it's a good idea, but when he gets out will he need that structure?

SAM: Let's cross that when we come to it. It's optimistic; we'll try our new medicine "Motivan"!

In contrast, what follows is an unusual interview in which the patient presented herself as responsible for her own actions.

■ The patient is an elderly woman who cries over the fact that she attacked her neighbor with an ice-pick.

SAM: Are you a God-fearing woman?

PATIENT: Yes.

SAM: Do you think God has forgiven you for this?

PATIENT: I suppose he has.

SAM: Do you think *you* can forgive you for this?

PATIENT: I'll try.

[Sam tells her gently that she was upset, that sometimes people do things they don't mean to. Later he says, "It's so rare to see remorse, I don't know what to do with it!"]

The unusual thing in this case was that the patient took responsibility for herself and wanted to be consistent in her behavior. She inspired admiration for fitting into the cultural ideal that we must give birth to ourselves as independent, productive, and consistent persons.

The medical atmosphere of the unit suggested that patients were too sick to work. But its isolation, regimentation, and efficiency implied the internalization of a discipline necessary for work. The staff singled out some patients as potentially capable, and for them the effort to make the unit "not a cradle" took the form of an insistence on responsibility. At times, this insistence was problematic. It raised doubts about the meaning of the work of the staff and about the kind of people they were. Was such behavior toward patients ultimately compassionate, or was it abuse?

III

There are rules. Codes, standards among civilized men. One doesn't cease behaving properly simply because one is entering a wilderness.
—ADMIRAL SCOTT in Terra Nova (Tally 1981:20)

There's no initiation either into such mysteries. He has to live in the midst of the incomprehensible, which is also detestable. And it has a fascination, too, that goes to work on him.
—JOSEPH CONRAD (1910)

I can't commute to a jungle, but I can come here.
—SAM WISHINSKI

Coming to terms with the "craziness" of administering the VIP treatment required that Ben, Sam, and to some extent the rest of the staff make sense of a practice that appeared profoundly inconsistent with the values expressed in the rest of their lives. Sam had a private practice in one of the city's better neighborhoods and was in training to become an analyst. Ben worked at other, less desperate hospitals. The students were idealistic about their potential to be helpful. Yet on the APU "the closer to patients the harder it was to be good." The staff had to face the possibility that personality could shift, maybe even unravel, in response to the peculiarities of the unit's demands (cf. Shweder and Bourne 1984).[2]

I was not the only outsider to be presented with the VIP treatment as a test of whether I could recognize this possibility. One visitor in particular became a paradigmatic example of outside incomprehension. Ben had discovered an emergency treatment center similar to the APU in the famous Big Hospital on the other side of the city. He came back quite excited. There, according to Sam:

Everyone wears white coats and they are scientific and they talk about data and they have computers. Their idea of brief treatments is like my idea when I first came here. I was going to shape this place up and have all the laboratory tests. Things would have to be so quick . . . and we would diagnose everything. Can you imagine trying to diagnose this guy [a not atypical patient we had just seen]? You could spend a year on him!

All their patients are voluntary, they all have insurance and—this is the big one—they [the staff] want the [diagnostic] tests because this is how they make money. They make much more money in the first three or four days. If they can do brief treatment they are getting the maximum value from each patient.

Ben was really impressed. He thought they might know things we don't know and thought they might also have come to some understanding . . . maybe that everyone doing brief hospitalization like this comes to some kind of inner change within themselves and that maybe this happened to them. So he came back and he said "We are not alone . . . I'm going to invite this guy [for a visit]:" So [Dr. K] came last Friday—very smart, well-dressed, scientific, the way a Big University faculty member should be. He generally was talking like a benevolent doctor except for the one lapse that patients are worth more during their first five days. Then he talked a little about how they use ECT [electroshock] therapy a lot; he could not believe we didn't have it. I was thinking [and I said to Ben later]—"That's a great idea, we would use the closet where we Kwell patients [use Kwell shampoo for lice] and while we're Kwelling them we could shock them too and the lice would jump off!" This shows how really demented, perverted, I've become here! But I censored that, I didn't say that. But then I told him the story of the VIP treatment to test his reaction. I said sometimes we wind up doing strange things on the unit because of the press of time and I wonder if you too have those sorts of experiences. He began looking a little uneasy and then he said "Ah yes! Confrontation!" See, he has to have an abstraction. Confrontation is OK, it's been written about, it's an accepted technique. And he said "Yes, yes, confrontation . . ." He repeated it two or three times. "Our nurses use plenty of confrontation, it's an accepted technique."

Later Ben took the visitor onto the unit. He reported that the doctor reacted with alarm. "It's so bleak," he said, "there are no pictures, I feel claustrophobic. No *wonder* no one wants to stay!"

This man reminded Sam once again of the dilemma raised in the play *Terra Nova*. At one point in the play, when Scott refuses to leave an injured man behind, Amundsen says to him disgustedly, "English, you don't even know who you are. You've learned every single rule, but not one dark corner of your own heart. You are the most dangerous kind of decent man" (1981:37). For Sam the question of decency was connected with what it meant to "do something that would seem harsh." He went on:

> *How often when we do something that seems benevolent it is merely for our-*
> *selves and not for the patient and how often the useful things we do for the*
> *patient are difficult, harsh things. I have to be comfortable in a situation in*
> *which it is impossible for me to be good.*
>
> *Here things are so muddled it's not clear whether when we do things that*
> *are nice we're doing things that are bad and whether when we do things that*
> *are bad it's because we're doing what we should. It's morally so murky here.*

In this recognition Sam and the rest of the staff differed from Admiral Scott. Scott was convinced to the end that he was doing right, unwilling to face the painful question of the relationship between morality and context. But in the "moral murk" of the APU it was clear to everyone that "doing bad" could not be avoided; does one begin to think of one-self as demented, or accept this shifting of the moral ground?[3]

One patient's stay on the unit coincided with a lecture Ben and Sam attended on the Holocaust, thus providing an uncomfortable extension of this theme. Frank Pankievich had been in the process of robbing an office when he fell asleep and was arrested. He was sent from jail for evaluation, much to everyone's initial amusement. But his presence was so malign that laughing at his incompetence seemed inappropriate. He had pale, unhealthy looking skin, sunken eyes, and was incredibly thin. The bones in his arms seemed about to poke through his skin. Sam talked about him in staffing:

SAM: He and I had an altercation. He proposes to go to Texas for the winter and pay [for the trip] with more robberies. He claims he's a more competent robber than we think! I said if he wanted treatment we would keep him a few days for meds but if he was going to play games we would send him back to jail. At that point he stopped talking to me.

RONNIE: He tried to call the public defender after that and then started acting really crazy.

SAM: I think he's crazy but incorporates it into a sociopathic routine. We could send him back to court and say that he's competent now but will be incompetent in a few days. Why would we want to drop charges?

LILLIAN: *Disgusting!* Send him back! Do y'all think he looks weird?

SAM: Well, he's a street person.

DUANE: And from New York!

SAM: He looks like a concentration camp victim, which influences people to drop charges and be good to this fragile soul.

This conversation contains an ironic twist, for Pankievich, like the APU staff, wanted to be thought competent even if what he did was unacceptable. Like other patients whom the staff felt might be competent (in several senses of the term) he was identified as a gameplayer, a man who had discovered the power of his own fragility.

Pankievich did come back a second time. "He was," said Lillian, "in restraints, like an animal, like a monster movie!" He continued to remind Sam of a concentration camp victim.

> *He ended up strapped to a bed and bathed in vomit, choking; he made us feel we were doing the evil we were so uncomfortable about. The stories about the holocaust which disturbed me most were about the kapos—Jews who would help the Nazis. I try to imagine, would I do that, would I rather die than do that? Yet here I am in a position as if I have prisoners here on the unit, and I sometimes room restrict them and they clearly regard me as [powerful]. It concretizes some basic conflicts I have, a coercive, sadistic side. I had an intuitive understanding of that guy.*

Pankievich hovered between being a monster and a victim. He was outstanding in his vulnerability, physical as well as mental. As Lillian said, "He was a *sick* man, very sick, gosh, was he sick!" Yet on the other hand he was manipulative, violent, someone toward whom all one's most "coercive" impulses could be acted out through the legitimate avenue of confinement. He embodied for staff the extreme alternatives implied by the patients' potential as prisoners. The coercive and abusive impulses he aroused made more real the possibility that they might be participants in an arrangement that was basically evil.

But Sam's coming to terms with his "Kapo" side also involved admitting the possibility that, as Amundsen suggests, the dark corners of his own heart might provide some of the more useful things he did.

> *Ben said early on that I would have to be comfortable with my own malevolence in order to survive here. The man from the Big Hospital said about the VIP treatment, "You know, it probably worked because you weren't really angry at the patient." He didn't want me to be angry and I thought the only way I could not be angry at that patient was if I didn't give a shit about him. The fact of the matter was I was angry at that patient and that was the most important thing he and I had going, that I cared enough to be*

angry and that I was sincere. If I had not been I don't think it would have worked.

In order to avoid experiencing the anger he [Dr. K] would have to avoid the whole thing altogether. He could be the most dangerous kind of decent man because in order to maintain his fragile sense of decency he would have to forego doing that sort of thing. He kept saying, "The way we do it [get them out fast] is we've got data coming in" and all the time, it was like a machine. People don't get angry and they use established techniques and they wear white coats. So the most dangerous kind of decent man is the kind of person I was when I came here.

The man from the Big Hospital, imaged as a medical technocrat, was the quintessence of heartless efficiency. He could be contrasted to the spontaneous, authentic response that cured the man given the VIP treatment. On the other hand Pankievich represented the possibility that such spontaneity could be carried too far, into a sadistic enjoyment of the patients' vulnerability as prisoners. Sam emphasized that he had changed through working on the unit and was no longer "decent," a "good boy," so intent on "seeking the Mother Theresa Award" that he was dangerous to his patients. Ben talked of his love of seedy places and of how he walked to the unit from his job at another hospital to "have time to metamorphose." But this capacity to change also carried an uncertainty about where the limits should be.

Sam used Conrad's story, the *Heart of Darkness* (1910), to talk about this question of limits. He compared the unit to the colonial wilderness that fascinates and perverts those who enter it.

What happens here is like the Heart of Darkness*; Kurtz in Europe is this civilized guy; you change his context and he becomes an utterly different person. His identity isn't what he thought, his boundaries aren't what they were. When I came here I had a particular identity as a psychotherapist— kind, helpful, etcetera. I retain that part of the day. In my suburban office I'm benevolent, mostly. Here, changing the context, I'm someone else.*

What particularly struck Sam about this parallel was the way the unit was hidden from outside authority in the matter of actual confrontation with patients. The invisibility of the staff went deeper than their ability to hide in strategies and forms; it extended to the effect they had on the patients. Sam compared this with his experience as a Peace Corps volunteer.

[While administering the VIP treatment] I had the feeling I had in the Peace Corps; I'm in the building with Bea and Anthony and all of them [the administration] but they don't want to know what goes on. I'm in an

outpost . . . and the patients don't pay me, they can't fire me. It's different from private practice. I say outrageous things to patients in private practice but it takes me a lot longer to get there, it's different.

Most of what happened between patients and the staff of the APU was within the limits of conventional practice—history-taking, the dispensing of medication, the routine physical care given by the nurses. We've already seen with the PPT and the mission memo that the administration attempted to maintain control over the details of the unit's operation. But Sam's belief that the administration preferred not to look was widely shared on the unit. The staff believed that some of what they did routinely would be shocking to outsiders and that occasional extremes (like the VIP treatment) were beyond the bounds of normal practice altogether. This conviction was shared with students, who often, as we have seen, developed a pride in their own adaptation to the unit's perspective.

This belief in a space of invisibility allowed the staff to feel that they could operate, in part, in the chinks and crannies formed by gaps in the routine surveillance of the unit. They defined these as spaces of freedom where they could invent unusual and spontaneous interventions with patients, though these interventions might also verge on a dangerous abuse of power. As Sam said about his experience in the Peace Corps, "It began to dawn on me that, my God, I was in a free universe, the despot of the place." The experiments that the staff carried out gained permission from books such as Farelly's *Provocative Therapy,* which suggest unusual or confrontive approaches to difficult patients.[4] But they were not planned and, from the staff's point of view, they arose unpredictably out of otherwise ordinary events. They took on an influence beyond their immediate effect because, like the story of the Judge and the VIP treatment, they threw into relief the dilemma of work on the unit. Ordinary intervention seemed to have no effect; perhaps "paradoxical" intervention, in which the patient was pushed in the direction he seemed to want to go, would yield better results.

MICHAEL JAMIESON CHANGES HIS MIND

> *One way to interrupt a client's pattern is to do something totally unexpected.*
>
> —BANDLER AND GRINDER (1982:18)

A homeless young man was admitted talking about suicide. He had slashed his wrists in the past and was a "wanderer" last hospitalized in another state. This was the initial discussion in staffing:

LILLIAN: He's been here before. He's the one that had that crazy hairdo last year—red, sticks up. He went upstairs before. They were glad not to get him this time.

SAM: He's been on Navane [an antipsychotic] in the past which helps, but hasn't had anything in the past few weeks. He had been staying with his brother, but he [the patient] beat him up. He does have a sister he says he could stay with.

ROBERT: Until he beats *her* up and then he can go back to his brother! [To medical student] He's yours, what do you think ought to be the goal?

STUDENT: Sober him up and hold him for a few days, then let him go. We can establish residence for him and consider day treatment.

Two days later, Michael was again discussed in staffing. Something had happened in the interval.

STUDENT: He isn't as crazy as he was.

SAM: He probably figured he had to get better! [To me, in an aside which soon becomes a kind of confession to the whole group] This was a paradoxical intervention. I asked him, "What can we do for you?" He said, "There's nothing." I said, "Just assuming you could have what you wanted, what would you like?" "I'd like you to put me to sleep [i.e., to kill him]." I than asked, "Well, how would you like us to do it?" "With a needle." "Do you have any other special requests before you go? Would you like a special meal before the end?"

Up to now, Sam said, it had been a run of the mill interview. But now Michael woke up. He said that he would like them to tell his brother he's sorry. Sam asked "At the funeral? Or where?" Michael said he wanted the staff to tell his brother how sorry he was, to write him a letter. At this point Sam said, "For tonight I'll give you an assignment. Write your brother, and write your funeral plans." Michael went off looking quite different. "Not exactly terrified, but like 'What is going on?'"

The next day he gave Sam the letter and a request that his brother visit him. That would take time, Sam said. Sam asked, "Am I to understand you don't want to die until then? We can put it off." Sam mailed the letter. [He says, "I checked on my malpractice insurance first!"]

This morning before staffing Jamieson informed Ronnie that he didn't want to die. He was looking pretty good, in good spirits.

SAM: Let's wait a few days.

STUDENT: To put him to sleep?

SAM: For him to talk to his brother. He has worked as a cook's assistant and does have job experience. Let's let him spend some time [here]. If he's not going to die, what is he going to do? This decision to live is a pretty heavy thing; he'll have to think about a job.

STUDENT: So what are you gonna do with him?

SAM: Wait.

RONNIE: God forgive us if we have to give a needle! A shot of anything. Do not consider Prolixin Decanoate for this man!

Sam talked about this incident later.

> *I told the story of Michael Jamieson [in staffing] because I felt unsure about doing it. I told Ben, gave him permission to say, "That's going too far." His reaction was "Ah, Bea's away for three weeks, we can do what we want." I told the medical student, looking for shock, but she was amused. I told my wife, and she laughed. Then she said, "Sam, you can't do that! Suppose he commits suicide to avoid being killed?" My concern is, what amount of suffering is this guy going through now as a result of what I've done? When I went through the intervention I wasn't unkind, I left it to him. I don't think he freaked out, but he was taking me seriously.*

> *I have misgivings about a lot of what I do. When you do these interventions there's nothing standard about them and* you're *alone; it's not like surgery with group support. [I ask, what about this group, the staff?] That's after the fact. And their enjoyment, maybe they felt disinhibited by my lack of inhibition. When I was doing it, I played it to the hilt;* I believed myself while I was doing it.

Five days later Jamieson was ready to be discharged. In staffing, someone had just referred to a previous patient as "one of the lucky ones."

SAM: Now we get to another lucky one—Michael Jamieson.

LILLIAN: I don't like him [lots of laughter]. Upstairs, too, they wouldn't take him. Everyone doesn't like him.

SAM: Is Michael still of a mind to live?

STUDENT: Yeah, for now. He plans to leave here, go to the mission, and go back to work for some shady character who gives him things to sell on the street. He says he can go to work for him and plans to move in with his sister after his check comes.

WALTER: Does she agree?

STUDENT: Yeah, after the first. He's basically bizarre . . . He says he gets crazy when he works.

LILLIAN and WALTER in unison: He's not the only patient who gets crazy when he works!

SAM: OK, he could go to the mission [this was before the mission memo]. Now let's consider our meds . . .

Though "no one was looking," it is clear that his experiment was (as Sam knew) tempered by the less flamboyant and more predictable work of the unit—medication and disposition. Obviously, however, the whole staff colluded with him in it, cooperating in conversations with Jamieson and listening with approval when Sam "confessed."

Unusual interventions like this made good stories. They provided the staff with opportunities to stress that they had a special understanding arising from their particular situation, and they contained an implicit defiance of the administration's agenda. The following brief and rather whimsical intervention soon gained a title: "The Secret Telegram." It was a telegram that had to be kept secret from the administration.

■ A patient had a fixed delusion of being a secret agent; he intervened in a knife fight, was arrested, and sent to the APU. The staff sent him a real telegram "from the agency" telling hem that he was to get an ordinary job in the community, "maintain a low profile," stop carrying weapons, and that his pay would come through DSS. He was thrilled to have finally heard from his control. He immediately began to look for a job, was discharged, and remained out of the hospital. Lillian said that when the telegram came, an administrator called her to sign for it; she was afraid that he would read it and find out what they had done.

Work on the APU raised two interrelated issues regarding the question of the self. The first had to do with consistency. The staff were uneasy about behavior that challenged their ordinary sense of self, a self that was, as for many Americans, assumed to be "an abstract entity independent of the social relations and contexts in which the self is presented in interactions" (Gaines 1982:182; cf. Schweder 1982; Geertz 1976).[5] The self that manifested in these interactions on the APU was context-dependent and seemed to form in response to situations. Sam stressed the intuitive, unpredictable aspect of himself that emerged in interactions such as that with Jamieson; he found himself spontaneously stepping out of the "run of the mill" expectations of both himself and the patient. In these interactions he "felt crazy" and yet he found that despite his misgivings he had touched on a potential in the patient that had remained out of sight as long as normal procedures were in place. In retrospect this appeared to be a kind of strategy, a form of competence as peculiar and context-specific as that involved in disposition, and even harder to explain.

But a second issue raised by these interactions was that they suggested a paradoxical relationship to the selfhood of patients. Paradoxical interventions involved an abandonment of decency, a refusal to adhere to rules, and a willingness to be spontaneous. Yet they were used to get patients to be decent—the good result, in the three examples I have given, was that the patient got (or looked for) a job. Allowing feelings to emerge—which was what effected the intervention—was precisely what the patients were being asked not to do.

Thus the mirroring involved in the relationship between the staff and patients was complex. The staff sometimes spoke of envying the patients their freedom to be crazy, and in these instances they seemed to take a little of that freedom for themselves. Yet they did so in the context of an emphasis on work and self-sufficiency in which the patients were expected to model themselves on the very self-control that had been set aside to make the point. Entry into the heart of darkness meant taking up the insider's perspective—the perspective of the patient—and playing along with "the native's point of view" even to the extent of acting on his fantasies. But the context was a space of discipline in which what counted—ultimately—was whether the patient could learn to work.

IV

The APU is no place for an idealist.

—Robert Naumann

We have looked for strange flowers here, in such an austere and ugly place.

—Sam Wishinski

Interventions like the VIP treatment and the offer to cooperate in Jamieson's suicide were self-conscious responses to the impossibility of being good. But they were rare. In day to day practice on the unit humor was a less drastic way to make the work possible. We have seen many examples of the humor of the staff, from their word-play in staffing to their mocking parodies of the standard language of psychiatry. The staff's humor was related to the issue of contextual identity; one way to align with the surroundings and yet maintain oneself as separate was to make a play on what was being done. For instance, in Sam's game of mental patient, every aspect of the patient's treatment is presented as an impossible double bind and the whole game is described from the patient's point of view, yet at the same time Sam creates a play on himself, the doctor, as the creator of the game (for instance, by his use of medical terminology ["organicity," "cirrhosis"]).

In order to be able to use humor, the staff had to accommodate to the unit's limitations. As with the issue of competence, they had to accept the futility of "rescue fantasies." But unlike disposition, which entailed a change in the definition of what could be done, humor entailed a change in what was seen. The staff member who developed what Barbara called "a certain levity" had learned to see the absurdity in situations that were also tragic and confusing. For students, this process involved a recognition of their limitations and the development of a willingness to laugh. One student, in a wonderfully confused passage, confessed that he didn't understand what made the unit funny but that he couldn't help but enjoy it.

> At first the unit was strange and alien. Well, it's a mental place so you think it's going to be crazy, dark, dirty, and hostile. But it's really not like that . . . you get a big kick out of working here. You know the patients by their bizarre behavior—like, "the one who's always grinning"—and it's satisfying to see them act that way. I don't know why. Maybe it's because you're not that way yourself. I get a charge out of seeing them do the things they do. I guess that's bad. You're not supposed to laugh at them, you're supposed to help. I guess you have to be there to see that it's valid and legitimate to laugh at them. I guess if you're involved in their care it's OK. That doesn't make sense, does it?

This student knows that his feelings would be unacceptable outside the unit—that "you're not supposed to laugh" at the patients. He sees that he has worked himself into a contradiction; the patients can be funny and somehow acceptable just as they are and yet still be under his care. He doesn't see what more experienced staff members made clear—that once the patients ceased being a challenge to their capacity to be good, they were free to enjoy them.

In the following episode, a student learned to associate limitation—the unit's and his own—with humor based on exaggeration and parody.

> We were in Screening dealing with a patient—he just got out of jail. He's staying at a mission, doesn't live anywhere. I'm sending him away, telling him to make an appointment, and he's saying he wants to make a phone call [to do it] but has no money. So I give him a quarter. Caldwell is in Screening and he says, Larry, you've got a big problem. I want you to spend all day with the patient helping him; it'll help you see how helpless you are. He

said to go and get the quarter back. OK, Caldwell said, why don't we make this a bank. *Naturally I refused. He insisted but I didn't go. He told the resident to take care of me, not to give me any more patients. Everyone on screening was laughing at this point and I started joking, playing on my own generosity, saying well, he can stay at my apartment . . . Later the patient tried to get carfare from me but I refused.*

For Ben, the student's offer of the quarter suggests a desire for omnipotence, a fantasy of providing for the patient that is likely to have no end. The lesson is contradictory: "helping the patient will help you see how helpless you are." Trying to help is exposed as not what it seems.[6] The student learns that joking can turn the situation around (for him and the other staff members, if not for the patient). Students might not come to recognize "the darkness in their own hearts" (perhaps that is a task for a later stage of life) but they discovered that humor could temper the harsh realities of work on the unit.

To say that the humor expressed in these situations was a safety valve, a way to deal with tension, is to trivialize it. The staff used humor to say something about themselves; through it they said, in a multitude of ways, we are *here* and no place else. Only from this angle, within this particular line of vision, can these things be seen as funny. They used humor to play on the tension between what was expected and ordinary and what was out of sight and extraordinary. Humor both created and celebrated intensity; in a minor way, it was like the expression of anger that Sam celebrated in the VIP treatment. It pushed the limits of what could be said or thought while acknowledging the limits of what could be done.

Humor also played on appearance. Many of the staff's jokes depended on reversals of expected categories or on exaggerations that stretched ordinary conventions. These were ways of playing on the contextual identity of the self, of deliberately creating the malleability that was otherwise so problematic. At their most extreme, they presented a carnivalesque vision of the unit as a place where "things are not as they seem, nor are they otherwise."

■ King James has been returning at ever shorter intervals. This time, when Sam sees him once again in the hall behind the window, he says, "My God, I'm hallucinating." He starts to "shake." "That's not, that *couldn't* be King James!" Feigning a man desperately struggling with psychosis, he reaches for the medicine cabinet and pours himself a "dose" of Haldol for his delusions. James, watching through the window, loves it.

■ Paul Goddard came into the unit doing an imitation of a patient which he had carefully prepared at home. He was dressed in colorful clothes and jumping

off the furniture, shouting "I'm the prophet James!" and "Here come the Kryp-
tonite beams!" He shows me the pages from the patient's chart which describe
him . . ." Bipolar affective disorder, mania, religious delusions . . ." Everyone is
laughing and the resident says, "We need a *male attendant* [what Paul is] for this
patient. [To Paul] They're gonna take away your keys and certify you!"

■   A hearing officer who had been coming to the center once a week for several
years was leaving. On his last day one of the medical students wore his oldest
shoes and a paper bag over his head, while another student "presented" him at
a hearing: "He's OK as long as he has this bag over his head, officer, but if you
take it off he goes wild and shouts all sorts of obscenities." The hearing officer
considered it a typical enough case until the joke was revealed, along with a cake
to celebrate his departure.

These episodes play on the possibility that the separation between the
staff and the patients is a fragile one. Through these inversions the
staff insist on the contingency and potential absurdity of their work,
reminding themselves and each other that "the 'reality' of appearance
is profoundly unreal" (Read 1980:165).[7]

The imagination that made this kind of humor possible also emerged,
at times, in the staff's acknowledgment of the patients' inner worlds. I
mentioned that the walls of the social workers' office were decorated
with magazine pictures of pretty outdoor scenes. Lillian, trying to explain her enjoyment of her work, said:

> *When someone is happily hallucinating it makes you happy. They have a*
> *license. Their craziness is something we can't do because we're too sensible.*
> *The beautiful pictures of the outside that we have up on our wall—they're*
> *inside them, too. Is it right to take it away from them?*

She didn't mean that she did not do what she could, for as we've seen
Lillian was practical and active in dealing with patients' problems. But
in this moment of reflection she suggests an image of the patients that
inverts the meanings usually assigned them, making of their craziness
something enviable. And, with inadvertent irony, she suggests that the
pictures inside the patients might match pictures of an outside world
beyond the city and beyond their reach.

I want to end with a brief conversation that contains many of the
recurring themes of this study. This patient was only on the unit for a
few days; he went back to jail and, ultimately, to the street. He seemed
to get what he wanted from the unit, yet he resisted efforts to persuade
him toward discipline and productivity. Medication helped and seemed
to offer some hope, but neither hope nor medication were pressed on
him. Perhaps, Sam said later, this brief interaction might someday influence him; if so, "It would be a hope for him and maybe for me; it would

vindicate my purpose here." But we never found out what happened to him.

Thornton was a young man arrested for disorderly conduct, with a history of mental illness and previous admissions to other hospitals. He was a pleasant looking man with sad eyes who had been living on the street for some time before he was arrested. Sam and a medical student interviewed him.

■ After a discussion of his medication, Thornton was asked about the possibility that he might hurt himself or others.

THORNTON: I'm not violent. I worry about today, living today. I'll cross the bridge of tomorrow when I come to it.

STUDENT: But you need to make provision for the future.

THORNTON: Well, that's putting the cart before the horse.

SAM: What do you think you need?

THORNTON: Group counseling once a month, no more often than that.

[I ask how he feels about taking the medication; he says that he wants peace of mind and finds freedom in meditation and walking.]

SAM: You put yourself down.

THORNTON: I keep a low profile. My goal in life is to live until I die.

[Sam tries to replay his history to him: when he takes medication he does OK, without it he breaks down. He fences, won't listen. He says he "wants to look at the fire and the rain."]

SAM: If we gave you meds you wouldn't be able to maintain your low profile [as a street person]. You might even get a job. Your wife might even come back.

THORNTON: I don't need a woman. I can do it with my own hand cheaper and easier.

SAM: That's like a sad song, I wake up with my love in my hand, not a woman in my arms. You've given up on everybody. When you want your chance, come back. Right now you want to stay crazy; of course, we don't want to mess up your life by making you sane.

THORNTON: I don't want to be what I'm not. I want to keep a low profile and low self-esteem, not show off among people. I'd rather be a bum than a damn king.

SAM: You could be in the middle.

THORNTON: I don't want to be neutral. It's one or the other.

SAM: OK, we'll send you back to court. You're competent, and we can't save you from being picked up.

As we left the room Thornton looked at us in surprise. Perhaps he had expected more argument.

Conclusion

I began my research on the Acute Psychiatry Unit by trying to respond to Anthony Giuliani's request that I look into the problem of aftercare. But I was soon caught up in the small, beleaguered world of the unit's staff. The staff insisted that the kinds of explanations I wanted weren't available and that I should beware of making things "look too concrete on paper." Instead of explaining, they told stories; instead of providing maps or diagrams, they made whimsical and idiosyncratic drawings.

Gradually I realized that the unit required a kind of balancing act. On one hand the staff maintained an awareness of what they regarded as the outside world. This world provided them with many kinds of guidelines and forms, from DSM III to laws governing patients' rights. On the other hand they were immersed daily in emerging situations that required immediate action. Often the forms did not fit the situation at hand. I began to shift my own perspective. The problem with aftercare was that it reified and located in the patient something that in fact was embedded in the practice of the staff. Though the staff sometimes used the vocabularies of institutional and community psychiatry, what they were doing did not fit into either model. They were practicing something else—getting patients out. They played Amundsen—pragmatic, hard-nosed, but able to get things done—to "regular" psychiatry's Scott.

After I left the APU I found that I could not get from my notes to a straightforward description of the unit. I kept getting entangled in the voices I had recorded, the commentary of the staff on their practice. Attempts to see through what they said to the "real" nature of the unit flattened out what had been, in the telling, funny, sad, and above all, inconclusive. The scene with which I began chapter 1, written by Sam some time after he left the unit, became symbolic for me of the staff's insistence that they tell their own story. Their story was about the interweaving of action and commentary that made the unit a site both of acquiescence to the institution's constraints and of a complex and strategic resistance.

This account has taken shape out of my effort to preserve the contradictory and multiple interpretations that the staff gave me. They were willing to expose the ambiguity that pervaded their actions and the emotions that informed and emerged from their decisions. At one point Lillian said of her reaction to my presence in staffing:

> *We got to the point where you could do with [your material] what you wanted, but we were going to tell you anyway, we didn't care what you wrote. We liked for you to see us functioning well or badly . . . sometimes I said mean things [about patients] but I thought, shit, she can write it down, that's OK. It was important that you saw all sides, it was realistic . . .*

The attempt to be true to "all sides" has proved more difficult than Lillian imagined. The realism of the unit consisted in a problematizing of all sides and a questioning of what, in its context, good or bad functioning might mean. My account cannot, in fact, be of "all sides," and I have instead allowed it to be as partial and as open to questions as the stories of the staff.

The APU staff represented themselves to me as unique, special, and different, aberrant villagers speaking from a part of psychiatry that they regarded as invisible. They drew my attention to the way the context of their work shaped their sense of competence, to the idiosyncratic solutions that emerged when they could not feel competent, and to the situated and singular quality of their understanding.

The staff's emphasis on efficiency developed out of and was shaped by the unit's properties as a disciplinary space pervaded by relations of power. The unit was modeled on the asylum with its apparatus of charts, schedules, and other techniques for making useful individuals. But with its mandate to keep people moving, the disciplinary aspects of this design were channeled into the one area where they could have the most effect: producing useful individuals might be impossible, but producing empty beds was not. In their push to get patients out, the staff resembled school children rushing against the clock to finish an exam or factory workers hurried by an assembly line speed-up (cf. Harvey 1989).

The challenge of this work was to make of efficiency an "included virtue" (Read 1980), something that marked the staff as competent in a way peculiar to this context. Paradoxically, the development of this situated competence could not take place entirely within the more visible aspects of the unit's operation. To employ the strategies and understandings that made them efficient the staff had to make use of the ways in which their work was hidden, turning the unit's starkness and the patients' difficulties into something other than what they seemed. When Ben said, "It's the attitude that we're unique that counts; who cares whether we really are or not?" he was pointing to the fact that practice on the unit depended on the staff's ability to make efficiency rewarding in ways that were uniquely theirs.

Thus, the unit's patients were treated as objects not simply because of the pressure on beds and time, but because responding efficiently to that pressure was the primary form that competence took among the staff. Disposition rewarded the staff with the mastery of a complex environment; what was "impossible" could be made into an intricate game with the playing itself a form of solace. The patients became the means to the end of producing empty beds, challenges to the staff's ability to negotiate a workplace that was perceived as a potential bottleneck.

But we have seen that while efficiency itself might be an acquiescence to the demands of strategy (while also making strategy rewarding) the staff simultaneously resisted these demands. Cultivating an underside to the unit's visible operations, they defined situations according to their understanding of the context. They made the unit a haven for some patients and unceremoniously threw others out; they expressed a great range of feelings, from anger, hatred, and bitterness to pity and compassion. They developed metaphors of "prison" and "home" to express the variable meanings arising from their position, creating a space of interpretation and commentary in whatever chinks of invisibility they could find. This elaboration of the unit's potential for contradicting itself gave the work an exuberance that escaped definition either by the orderliness of abstract architecture or the disorderliness of patients.

The APU staff made a point about their uniqueness that can be expanded, not to an assumption that the APU was (or was not) different from other clinics, but to a more general understanding of the nature of situated knowledge. The staff spoke from a place, a position, that was specific and local, grounded in the exigencies of a particular set of constraints and possibilities. What they spoke about was their own situated understanding, not likely to be duplicated elsewhere, of the contradictions emerging from their spot in time and space. This kind of knowledge is what Foucault calls "subjugated knowledge."

> . . . by subjugated knowledges one should understand . . . a whole set of knowledges . . . beneath the required level of cognition of scientificity . . . it is through the re-emergence of these low-ranking knowledges . . . (such as that of the psychiatric patient, of the ill person, of the nurse, of the doctor—parallel and marginal as they are to the knowledge of medicine) . . . that criticism performs its work. (1980:98)

These knowledges are "particular, local, regional . . . incapable of unanimity." They are plural and fragmentary. They are the knowledges of the aberrant villager, the mental health worker, the public psychiatrist, even the frustrated administrator, who speak to us from an unconscious of psychiatry where they are "opposed by everything around them." As Ben said when he threw a patient out, "I knew it was the right thing to do, but it didn't fit into the well-intentioned perspective."

The situated knowledge of the APU staff had three components. The first was the knowledge of how to situate the "knowledge of medicine" within the reality of practice. The staff knew how to make diagnosis and medication serve efficiency and how to use the language provided by medicine and community psychiatry in the context of the unit's dilemmas. Renee, for example, was asked to situate the textbook definition of the borderline patient in the context of Mr. A's rage and Sam's recommendation to "hold his nose until he becomes a purple elephant." In this sense all knowledge is situated knowledge, and the staff played on the humor to be found in recognizing this fact.

The second component of the staff's situated knowledge was their resistance to the knowledge of medicine and the discipline of the unit. This resistance was oblique, not opposed as "truth" to some sort of singular oppressive power, but developed at an angle to the expected definitions of situations. The staff were cunning, devious, and actively ignorant in moving among the threads of power on the unit, taking advantage of areas of invisibility. They redefined their work to emphasize its contradictions; they redefined patients into categories of their own making; they resisted administrative rules. Their situated knowledge involved a double vision, keeping in sight what was expected while looking, as well, at what was specific, partial, and visible only from where they stood (cf. Haraway 1988).

Finally, the staff's situated knowledge included a self-conscious awareness that it *was* a situated knowledge. Mostly spoken, subject to changes of all kinds, it was recognized by them to be homemade and fragile. They urged me to write it down partly, I think, for that reason. Perhaps this self-consciousness is a characteristic of such knowledges, since they are formed in an awareness of a larger context and are to some extent a deliberate commentary on being different and set apart. But it was a paradox of work on the unit that the task was made bearable by self-conscious and sometimes comic commentary.

The knowledge of the APU staff was ephemeral and open-ended. We cannot find in it any easy solutions to the problems they were charged with managing. But by understanding that theirs was a situated knowledge, taking its shape from the intricacy of a specific practice and incapable of abstraction from it, we can begin to see "the arbitrariness of institutions" and perhaps find a starting point for criticism.

Afterword

It changes so fast, from one second to the next. Are you going to put that in your book?

—NANCY ALTMAN

When I left the APU after two years of study, the unit was in the process of a major change. Sam had left for a job in another city, and Ben was about to become director of an emergency unit in a nearby general hospital. Remaining staff members complained that the unit was not processing patients fast enough and was becoming "clogged up" and boring.

I returned for a visit two years later to find little that seemed familiar. The day room had been moved to the area formerly occupied by Screening; the old day room was a staff lounge. Plants in the lobby and pictures on the walls gave evidence of the success of Giuliani's efforts to soften the institutional environment. Most of the staff members I knew had left; Lillian worked in another hospital, and Sally was planning her retirement. I sensed that the unit I had studied was closed.

When I talked with Anthony Giuliani, he told me that the APU was taking a different approach to patients. They still stayed for short periods, but their care was better. "It's not so funny there now," he said, "but it's more responsible. Ben and Sam went too far."

Lillian told me about some of the patients I had known. The Judge was still at the state hospital, "doing fine." Fischer came in and out intermittently as always; he was "just the same."

Keith was dead. He had seemed happy at State Hospital until, without warning, he hanged himself in a nearby park. "Everyone," said Lillian, "took it hard. We had got used to him, he was 'just Keith.'" She repeated several times how surprising Keith's death had been. "It just shows," she said, "that we don't know everything."

Notes

Introduction

1. Verbatim passages in this account were mainly recorded in the form of notes.
2. The idea of asking for drawings came to me after reading Gaines' paper on psychiatrists' models of treatment (1979). My request was extremely open-ended, resulting in a wide variety of interpretations by the staff.
3. I am indebted to E. V. Daniel for this phrase.

Starkness Was Everywhere

1. An acutely psychotic patient, especially one who was fairly young, was believed by the staff to be far more likely to recover than an older, chronically ill patient. Thus alarming symptoms were no measure of the true difficulty involved in treating a patient.
2. The unit's seclusion rooms could be converted into patient rooms when there was a shortage of beds.
3. Some of those named are composites.
4. Ellen Dwyer notes similar ambiguities in the role of hospital workers in the nineteenth century; they were "close to the bottom of the asylum work hierarchy" and had "the heaviest work responsibilities in the asylum but little formal power" (1987:164). Similar issues of low pay and close association with patients seemed to be involved.
5. Goffman (1961) resembles Foucault (especially 1979) in his disinclination to include subjectivity in his account of the strategies involved in asylum life. But it is not clear to what extent he recognized the relationship between the structure of the institution and the consciousness of both patients and staff.
6. In his description of the "underside" of the asylum Goffman (1961) also describes the ways in which the patients and staff use the margins and hiding places available in the organization and space of the institution.
7. Starr points out that this loose coordination of authority is characteristic of hospitals (1982:178).

We Discharge in Ten Days

1. This remark comes from Dostoyevsky's Grand Inquisitor (*The Brothers Kara-mozov*), quoted whimsically by Sam.

2. The staff recognized that labeling a person mentally ill could be detrimental to her life; for example, they tried to discharge patients who had jobs and did not want their employers to know they were hospitalized. However, the theory that labeling is a primary factor in causing (or constructing) mental illness (see, e.g. Szaz 1961) seemed far from the realities of the unit's work.

3. There are several handbooks of emergency psychiatry addressed specifically to workers in emergency rooms; see, e.g., Cumming (1983) and Soreff (1981).

4. Major psychiatric medications include neuroleptics that act on the symptoms of psychosis (Prolixin, Mellaril), lithium for manic-depressive illness, and the antidepressants. Some of these medications have side effects such as akathesia and tardive dyskinesia that influence patients' willingness to continue taking them even when they alleviate their psychotic symptoms. Estroff points out that these side effects often have profound effects on patients' social lives. See Estroff (1985), Rhodes (1984), Klerman (1977).

5. Some recent writers on mental illness have discussed the connection between symptoms of mental illness and unemployment. Warner studied the rates and symptomatology of schizophrenia and found a correlation with rates of unemployment and the subjective reactions of men to unemployment (1985). Almost all the patients who came into the APU were unemployed; we will see in chapter 7 that the staff drew some connections between intention, work, and illness. But no one on the APU mentioned unemployment as a cause of mental illness; if anything, they saw the causal relation pointing in the opposite direction.

6. This submarine metaphor contrasts with the one provided by the nurse in chapter 1 who highlights the control room. The APU may have lent itself to submarine metaphors because of its physical position in a dark and slightly subterranean part of the hospital.

7. The APU staff talked of their emphasis on discharge as unusual and, in fact, their single-mindedness in "aiming toward separation" contrasted with the other units in the hospital. But in a utilization review prepared by the administration it is apparent that the center as a whole experienced the pressure of numbers:

    > As we are responsible for treating large numbers of patients, it is necessary that we give consideration to the efficiency, as well as the effectiveness, of our treatments.

8. Starr points out that the orientation toward colleagues (rather than clients) that defines professionalism violates the rules of a market economy: "There are no relations of dependency in an ideal market" (1982:23). Ben's analogy can be read as an insistence on autonomy and independence developing out of a breakdown of clear institutional arrangements; in other words, the APU staff are entrepreneurs of aftercare in the wake of deinstitutionalization.

9. The APU social workers often, but not always, said "clients." The rest of the staff said "patients."

10. Bachrach discusses the euphemistic vocabulary that characterizes psychiatry; it is obvious from her essay itself that there are few straightforward words available in this field!

> . . . *semantic games seem to permeate all aspects of service delivery for mentally disabled people . . . we often use catchwords, buzzwords, euphemisms, slogans and metaphors to minimize the complexity of the problems . . . (1985:15)*

11. The notion of "dangerous to self" could be extended to patients who were judged unable to care for themselves adequately. The question of dangerousness to others involved the staff in predictions about the future that seemed to them highly problematic. Shah writes that:

> *It is . . . difficult to discern how this [legal] link between mental illness and dangerous behavior came about and why it continues to be maintained with such . . . zeal . . . to protect the community against dangerous individuals, the state typically uses its police powers. However, the criminal process is invoked after the individual has engaged in some harmful act . . . [1982:276]*

The hearing process, the documentation of suicide risk, and the other preventive aspects of their work involved the APU staff in decisions based on *potential* "harmful acts."

12. The hearing was sometimes what Goffman calls a ritual of mortification (1961) in which the patient's failures were exposed to public scrutiny. For example, a relative might be called and asked for a description of the patient's behavior that would be heard by everyone in the room.

13. The satellite clinics complained that the APU sometimes released patients from the hospital too soon, before they were able to manage independently.

14. In chapter 6 I discuss in more detail the implications of discharging patients to the mission.

15. See Warren (1981) and Scull (1979) for critical discussions of the economics involved in the development of boarding homes.

16. The University was shifting to a more biological orientation during the time of this study; however, for many of the psychiatrists working at the Douglass Center the analytic perspective in which they had been trained carried the most prestige.

The Game of Hot Shit

1. In *Terra Nova* Amundsen insists that "There is only one way to live here, one only! Everything is a *tool* . . . if it breaks down you throw it away and march on! It's brutal, yes! . . . But anything else is sentimental and will kill you!" (Tally 1981:37)

2. Good suggests that there is, on the one hand, the question of physician competence itself, which assumes "competence as an empirical reality," and, on the other, the symbolic domain of the "discourse on competence." Like her, I am interested in the "constitutive" aspects of a particular discourse, not with the question of whether the practice of the APU was "competent" (1985:249–250).

3. See chapter 7 for several examples of the "relabeling" of patients' situations.

4. Sam assigned the "case management" of patients on an ad hoc basis. In this case Walter was particularly qualified because of his role as alcoholism counselor.

5. For discussions of uncertainty in medicine and psychiatry, see, e.g., Fox (1963), Light (1980), and Coser (1979). Light points out that uncertainty in psychiatry involves a "scramble for techniques of control" (1980:282), one of which is a commitment to the "approach" of a particular therapeutic theory or technique. On the APU, theoretical perspectives in psychiatry seemed less important than the shared focus on the rapid movement of patients; this could be considered, in Light's terms, the ideology that kept uncertainty at bay. Its fragility is apparent in many conversations recorded in this book.

6. Rittenberg (1985) presents a case that resembles this one in coalescing clinical staff around a particular point of view. Such cases become "projects of action" (Rittenberg 1985; Schutz 1967) that emerge from routine practice and remain in memory as representations of problematic aspects of the work.

History Modifies Our Fantasies

1. Jones points out that psychiatric history has a cyclical pattern marked by periods of enthusiasm for reform followed by troughs of disinterest (1979: 553).

2. Accounts of the history of psychiatric institutions are complicated by questions about the relationship between European and American developments. Foucault focuses on the history of confinement in Europe and the development in the nineteenth century of an emphasis on self-restraint in the place of physical coercion (1973). Rothman writes about the asylum in America as an image of order and restraint, but does not emphasize its European origins (1971). For my purposes, the coherence in the design of asylums and the parallels in notions of restraint on both sides of the Atlantic are more important than the historical differences between the two continents. See Baruch and Treacher (1978) for a discussion of some of the difficulties in writing psychiatric history.

3. See Starr (1982:169) for a discussion of the difference between mental and general hospitals in America and Scull (1981) for a description of the professional development of asylum doctors in England. Starr points out that mental hospitals developed by getting bigger and remaining outside towns and cities, whereas general hospitals multiplied in number and remained in populated areas.

4. See Bachrach (1976), Estroff (1981, 1985), Jones (1979), Busfield (1986), Mollica (1983), and Scull (1977) for a variety of perspectives on the process and results of deinstitutionalization. Jones points out that the community mental health center movement in the United States generated innovative approaches to deinstitutionalization and community treatment. However, the financial pressures that followed the initial phase meant that the planned network of support services often did not materialize. Scull sees this as the inevitable result of an adherence, on the part of the state, to a program of cost reduction.

> If the program for decarcerating the mentally ill was to live up to rhetorical claims about its being undertaken for the ex-patient's welfare, . . . aftercare facilities would have had to be extensively present; but this would have been extremely costly, and if the program was to realize financial savings they had to substantially absent. They are absent. (Scull 1984:142)

5. The difference between these two perspectives is sometimes described as a controversy between reformists and revisionists. A helpful guide to the issues can be found in Cohen and Scull (eds.), *Social Control and the State* (1983), particularly the essays by Ignatieff, Scull, Ingleby, and Rothman. The reform/revision debate is marked by a degree of hostility on both sides (Scull 1983:118) that probably reflects the closeness of the issues to fundamental concerns in Western culture about freedom, intentionality, and progress. Writers on this subject tend to use different vocabularies depending on their perspective: for the revisionists, patients are "mad" or "deviant" rather than "mentally ill" and they are subjected to "decarceration" rather than "deinstitutionalized." The staff of the APU combined these vocabularies in their everyday talk, adjusting them to the specific contexts of their practice.

6. Estroff (1981, 1985, 1988), Bachrach (1976, 1987), Klerman (1977), Sheehan (1983), Landy (1982), Scheper-Hughes (1981, 1982) for example, discuss, from different perspectives, the question of chronicity and the ways in which psychiatric patients are caught up in difficult issues of identity and functioning. Hopper and Hamburg (1984) and Hopper (1988) discuss the causes of homelessness and dislocation in the inner city and the ways in which psychiatric labeling can function to conceal economic and political issues. Scull (1981a, 1981b, 1984) and Warren (1981) point to the economic aspects of the closing down of costly state hospitals and the development of entrepreneurial "community" care.

7. Foucault argues that practices, language, and historical context are intertwined in ways that make causal explanation problematic and that the larger issue in the debates about psychiatry is the relationship between subject and object in our culture (1973, 1980, 1983).

8. In an article written in 1973 for a book on community mental health a psychologist compares the attitude needed in a university with that appropriate to community work:

> Another hangup that we professionals have is our tendency to structure our lives and fill our curriculum as if our pieces of knowledge were bits of honey in a beehive. We so preempt our lives with our definitions of professional practice that we allow little room for picking up a piece of the action . . . The community psychologist needs free hours . . . Community events . . . represent our laboratory . . . (Kelley 1973:181)

In retrospect, Ben sees both the innocence and arrogance of this combination of scientism ("our laboratory") with an assumption that "pieces of the action" were just waiting to be "picked up" by the community psychologist: "I had my psycho-social period then."

9. Wellin et al. 1987 describe the combination of approaches that resulted in the creation of psychiatric emergency services.

10. The fact that Ben (and Sam) "could always get another job" probably contributed to their flexible approach to work on the unit. See Light (1980:320–321) for a concise discussion of the motivations of young psychiatrists involved in public psychiatry.

11. The confusion expressed here about "being all things to all people" can be seen as an aspect of a larger problem of normalization and medicalization in which the hospital participates. If definitions of the normal provide the standard against which ever-expanding areas of illness or deviance can be

"known," then "outreach" programs like community psychiatry are not different in kind from institutional practice (Foucault 1978, 1979; Arney and Bergen 1984). Both the community programs and the hospital's open door suggest a willingness to serve an ever-enlarging array of problems (cf. Kovel 1980).

12. The staff attributed some of their current loss of freedom to the increased numbers of court-ordered patients on the unit. Because it was small and short-term, the unit had become a primary evaluation center for court-ordered patients. It is also likely that there were more court-ordered patients in the system as a whole as it became more difficult to commit patients to the hospital and as patients found it more difficult to admit themselves.

13. Light reviews the work of Kahn-Hat on the attitudes of psychiatrists to their work. She found that "psychiatrists did not deny the alienating conditions of their work . . . instead they converted them into sources of satisfaction" (Light 1980:323, quoting Kahn-Hat).

Whatever Takes Less Writing

1. Diagnosis is a controversial subject within psychiatry. See Kleinman for a discussion of the interpretative aspects of psychiatric diagnosis (1988) and Fabrega for a discussion of issues of classification involved in diagnosis (1987). Ingleby claims that the problem rests in the natural science claims of psychiatry to objectively describe as facts (entities) what are in fact culturally and socially determined behaviors (1982:33). Many observers have noted that psychiatric diagnoses "label" patients in ways that medical diagnoses do not; one "has" a medical disease, while one "is" a psychiatric diagnosis (Estroff 1988; Szas 1961). While diagnosis is considered unimportant from a psychoanalytic perspective, Light notes that psychiatric residents use the APA labels to describe patients even when they also say that these labels "mean nothing" because they only label the "leading style or symptom" of the patient. Thus "the terms become an essential, telegraphic vocabulary for the professional staff" (1980:176–177).

2. American Psychiatric Association, 1980. This reference volume is revised periodically to reflect changes in psychiatric opinion; on the APU its categories were usually treated in practice as fixed and absolute, though an example of criticism is discussed in this chapter.

3. APU residents and medical students sometimes commented that when they first began their rotation they suddenly became aware of how much "pathology" was "walking around on the streets." But these people were not (yet?) "cases."

4. One aspect of this independence was an unusual freedom to "practice" interviewing techniques. One student who got interested in organic disorders said, "Since I picked up on this organic testing I've been practicing it on everybody whether they need it or not."

5. The use of the chart to objectify and "stand in" for the patient has been noted by many observers of hospitals, for instance Goffman (1961) or Szaz (1961). Foucault's analysis is more subtle than the social control perspective assumed in most of these accounts (which consider the charting of patients a function of their deviance rather than a mechanism that "normalizes" everyone involved).

6. In the writing of psychiatric diagnoses, "where there are no signs of pathology, the patient is described in such a way as to leave open the question of undisclosed pathology" (Light 1980:163).

7. "Borderline" is a much-debated diagnostic category that describes "instability in a variety of areas, including interpersonal behavior, mood and self-image . . . frequently there is impulsive and unpredictable behavior" (APA 1980:321).

8. See Light (1980:186–206) for a discussion of the various techniques used in case conferences to expose or outwit the "defenses" of the patient.

9. Sudnow (1963) writes about the "normal crimes" that structure the work of a D.A.'s office; Light notices the same tendency to focus on "normal pathology" in the psychiatric hospital (1980). See also Mizrahi (1986:92).

10. The focus on "interesting" pathology noted by Mizrahi (1986) and others for the general hospital seemed less important on Emergency Services, perhaps because the large numbers of patients ensured a constant flow of "interesting" cases.

11. Arney and Bergen argue that "objectify" needs to be qualified with an understanding that "medicine has changed its understanding of what kind of object the patient is" (1984:50). Though I feel they are too totalizing in their view that systems theory has entirely remade the medical perspective, their analysis is helpful in understanding the APU's response to the charting of patients.

12. The student is referring to the use of lithium, which is sometimes effective in eliminating the symptoms of manic-depression without affecting the patient's personality.

13. This issue of emotional closeness/distance is pervasive in physicians' accounts of their work, for example in accounts of medical school and residency (e.g., Konner 1987), and in accounts of training and practice (e.g., Hahn 1985; Fox and Harold 1963).

14. See, e.g., Stamm, for a discussion of countertransference in hospital treatment. He defines "countertransference acting out" as "the staff members taking . . . action toward a patient based on a feeling, impulse, attitude or fantasy . . ." (1987:7) and quotes Main (1957) to the effect that "patients who do not get well . . . stir the most primitive reactions within treaters." See also Devereux (1980) for a discussion of the psychological aspects of diagnosis.

15. This is a crude version of the "repair" metaphor implied in the medical model; its ambiguousness in the context of psychiatry is discussed by, e.g., Goffman (1961) and Siegler and Osmund (1976).

16. Grob notes that in the American asylums of the early nineteenth century records were kept chronologically in large books so that information about any one patient was scattered in many different places. Adolph Meyer, a Swiss immigrant, began his new job as superintendent at Worcester State in the 1890s by changing this tradition:

    Meyer succeeded in getting the hospital to keep individual records in a single folder. Thus all material pertaining to any patient—even those readmitted—was easily accessible. (1983:83)

17. The patient's privacy was felt to be exposed in the chart in a way that it was not in personal contact; while I was free to talk to patients or sit in on interviews, I had to have special permission to see patients' charts.

18. Lentricchia goes on to say that "Foucault has not produced convincing evidence that Bentham's demonic ideal is our only social reality" (1988:82). In fact, I think, Foucault does not argue that the ideal is the only social reality, only that it profoundly shapes a social reality that also struggles against it. This is clearer in his later work than it is in *Discipline and Punish* (1979).

19. As Mizrahi points out, this replacement of the patient by the chart can happen whether or not the chart is an "accurate" representation of the patient's situation (1986). See also Goffman (1961).

20. Arney and Bergen (1984) relate this development to the influence of systems theory; the ecological model, in their view, provides a rationalization for extending the normalizing function of medicine. See note 14, above.

21. For discussions that make explicit the aspect of visibility in charting see Mumford (1970:152) and Bosk (1979:78–79).

Like Migrating Birds

1. Estroff points out that the dependence of the chronic patient has as its obverse the dependence of those who care for them: "Who indeed is dependent on whom? Literally hundreds of thousands of producing/labeling persons depend upon dependent persons for their livelihood" (1988:27). From this perspective, it was in the interests of APU staff to emphasize the "overwhelming needs" of their patients, though in fact they did not always do so. The usefulness to the administration of an "overload" of patients is directly indicated, later in this chapter, by Giuliani.

2. This patient was taking lithium for manic-depression and was expressing, in the student's view, a reluctance to "come down" from an enjoyable, if delusional, manic state.

3. Of course I had no actual or legal responsibility for Keith; I did not make decisions regarding him, make suggestions to him, or write in his chart.

4. This account is of Keith as he was understood by staff and as he presented himself on the unit. I do not explore his life outside, or the meaning that events might have had to him outside the context of the unit; for example, I do not know whether he really had the kittens he describes. For accounts of patients' perspectives on repeated hospitalization see, e.g., Sheehan (1983), Estroff (1985), and Scheper-Hughes (1981).

5. As an anthropologist with an interest in ritual, I was the perfect observer for this scene. Perhaps it would not have happened had I not been there.

6. This is a good expression of the kind of bind described by Estroff for the outpatients she studied (1985); Keith cannot expect care—from his mother or from the hospital—if he "learns not to be stupid."

7. Kim Hopper points out that labeling the homeless as deviant is a way to mystify the causes of their situation (1988); in this case the patient is eager to cooperate, given the alternatives to hospitalization.

It Is Impossible To Be Good

1. Most of the patients discussed in this chapter were regarded by the staff as suffering from "character disorder" rather than psychosis. They were considered tougher and more in need of "limits" than more acutely disturbed patients.

2. Much has been written about the socialization of physicians (see Light 1980, chap. 15, for a discussion of the issues; he insists, rightly, I think, on the dynamic quality of the process). The APU staff were already socialized into professional roles that precluded some of what they describe in this chapter; I believe that the issue, for them, was primarily about the malleability of identity rather than a concern for their image as professionals.

3. An article by Searles entitled "The 'Dedicated Physician' in Psychotherapy and Psychoanalysis" was referred to by Ben and Sam as an argument for "bad" really being good. Searles suggests that too much dedication on the part of the therapist is bad for schizophrenic patients: "In general, if the patient's illness is causing more suffering to the therapist than to the patient, then something is wrong" (1967:131).

4. See also Haley (1984). Farelly says of provocative therapy, "The therapist sides with . . . the negative half of the client's ambivalence toward himself . . . He takes the 'crooked' part of the script . . . thereby provoking the client to take the more rational . . . portion" (1978:57).

5. Context-dependent selfhood, in which "self . . . varies from interaction to interaction" (Gaines 1982:183) is described by Gaines for Mediterranean cultures and by Schweder for India (1982).

6. See Light (1980, chap. 14) and Sharaf and Levinson (1964) for discussions of the issue of omnipotence in psychiatry.

7. Kenneth Read, in an ethnography of a homosexual tavern (1980), provides a brilliant discussion of the way a "community of believers" uses humor to construct an elaborate parody of the assumptions of a straight world in which their participation can only be indirect.

Bibliography

AMERICAN PSYCHIATRIC ASSOCIATION
  1980   *Diagnostic and Statistical Manual of Mental Disorders,* 3d ed. Washington, D.C.: APA.

ARNEY, WILLIAM RAY, and BERNARD J. BERGEN
  1984   *Medicine and the Management of Living: Taming the Last Great Beast.* Chicago: University of Chicago Press.

BACHRACH, LEONA L.
  1976   *Deinstitutionalization: An Analytical Review and Sociological Perspective.* National Institute of Mental Health, DHEW Publication No. (AIM) 76–351.
  1985   *Slogans and Euphemisms: The Function of Semantics in Mental Health and Mental Retardation Care.* Austin, Tex.: Hogg Foundation for Mental Health.
  1987   *Leona Bachrach Speaks: Selected Speeches and Lectures.* New Directions for Mental Health Services #35. San Francisco: Jossey-Bass.

BANDLER, RICHARD, and JOHN GRINDER
  1982   *Reframing: Neuro-Linguistic Programming and the Transformation of Meaning.* Moab, Ut.: Real People Press.

BARUCH, GEOFF, and ANDREW TREACHER
  1978   *Psychiatry Observed.* London: Routlege and Kegan Paul.

BELLAH, ROBERT N., RICHARD MADSEN, WILLIAN N. SULLIVAN, ANN SWIDLER, and STEVEN M. TIPTON
  1985   *Habits of the Heart.* Berkeley, Los Angeles, London: University of California Press.

BERMAN, MARSHALL
  1982   *All That Is Solid Melts Into Air: The Experience of Modernity.* New York: Simon and Schuster.

BOSK, CHARLES L.
  1979   *Forgive and Remember: Managing Medical Failure.* Chicago: University of Chicago Press.

BOURDIEU, PIERRE
  1977   *Outline of a Theory of Practice.* Trans. Richard Nice. Cambridge: Cambridge University Press.

BUSFIELD, JOAN
  1986   *Managing Madness*. London: Hutchinson.

CAUDILL, WILLIAM
  1958   *The Psychiatric Hospital as a Small Society*. Cambridge: Harvard University Press.

CLIFFORD, JAMES
  1986   "Introduction: Partial Truths" in *Writing Culture: The Poetics and Politics of Ethnography*, ed. J. Clifford and G. Marcus. Berkeley, Los Angeles, London: University of California Press.

COHEN, S., and A. SCULL
  1983   *Social Control and the State: Historical and Comparative Essays*. Oxford: Martin Robertson.

COMAROFF, JEAN
  1985   *Body of Power, Spirit of Resistance: The Culture and History of a South African People*. Chicago: University of Chicago Press.

CONRAD, JOSEPH
  1910   *The Heart of Darkness and The Secret Sharer*. New York: New American Library.

COSER, ROSE LAUB
  1979   *Training in Ambiguity: Learning Through Doing in a Mental Hospital*. New York: Free Press.

CUMMING, ROBERT G.
  1983   *Casebook of Psychiatric Emergencies: The 'On Call' Dilemma*. Baltimore: University Park Press.

DEVEREUX, GEORGE
  1980   *Basic Problems in Ethnopsychiatry*. Chicago: University of Chicago Press.

DREYFUS, HUBERT, and PAUL RABINOW
  1983   *Michel Foucault: Beyond Structuralism and Hermeneutics*, 2nd ed. Chicago: University of Chicago Press.

DWYER, ELLEN
  1987   *Homes for the Mad*. New Brunswick, N.J.: Rutgers.

EDWARDS, REM BLANCHARD
  1982   *Psychiatry and Ethics*. Buffalo, N.Y.: Prometheus Books.

ESTROFF, SUE E.
  1981a "Psychiatric Deinstitutionalization: A Sociocultural Analysis." *Journal of Social Issues* 37(3):116–132.
  1985   *Making It Crazy: An Ethnography of Psychiatric Clients in an American Community*, 2d ed. Berkeley, Los Angeles, London: University of California Press.
  1988   "Identity, Disability and Schizophrenia: The Problem of Chronicity." Paper prepared for Wenner-Grenn Conference #106, Analysis in Medical Anthropology.

FABIAN, JOHANNES
  1983   *Time and the Other: How Anthropology Makes Its Object*. New York: Columbia University Press.

FABREGA, HORACIO
    1987   "Psychiatric Diagnosis: A Cultural Perspective." *The Journal of Mental Disorders* 175(7):383–394.

FARELLY, FRANK, and JEFF BRANDSMA
    1978   *Provocative Therapy.* Fort Collins, Colo.: Shields Publishing Company.

FAVRET-SAADA, JEAN
    1980   *Deadly Words: Witchcraft in the Bocage.* Trans. Catherine Cullen. Cambridge: Cambridge University Press.

FOUCAULT, MICHEL
    1973   *Madness and Civilization: A History of Insanity in the Age of Reason.* Trans. Richard Howard. New York: Vintage Books.
    1975   *The Birth of the Clinic: An Archaeology of Medical Perception.* Trans. A. M. Sheridan Smith. New York: Vintage Books.
    1978   *The History of Sexuality. Vol. 1: An Introduction.* Trans. Robert Hurley. New York: Pantheon Books.
    1979   *Discipline and Punish: The Birth of the Prison.* Trans. Alan Sheridan. New York: Vintage Books.
    1980   *Power/Knowledge: Selected Interviews and Other Writings.* Ed. Colin Gordon. New York: Pantheon Books.
    1983   "The Subject and Power." In *Michel Foucault: Beyond Structuralism and Hermeneutics,* 2nd ed. Ed. Hubert Dreyfus and Paul Rabinow. Chicago: University of Chicago Press.

FOUCAULT, MICHEL
    1984   "Polemics, Politics and Problemizations: An Interview." In *The Foucault Reader,* ed. Paul Rabinow. New York: Pantheon.

FOX, RENEE
    1974   *Experiment Perilous: Physicians and Patients Facing the Unknown.* Philadelphia: University of Pennsylvania Press.

FOX, RENEE, and HAROLD LIEF
    1963   "Training for 'Detached Concern' in Medical Students." In *The Psychological Basis of Medical Practice,* ed. H. I. Lief, V. F. Lief, and N. Lief. New York: Harper and Row.

GAINES, ATWOOD D.
    1979   "Definitions and Diagnoses: Cultural Definitions of Psychiatric Help-seeking and Psychiatrists' Definitions of the Situation in Psychiatric Emergencies." *Culture, Medicine and Psychiatry* 3(1):381–418.
    1982   "Culture Definitions, Behavior and the Person in American Psychiatry." In *Cultural Conceptions of Mental Health and Therapy,* ed. A. J. Marsella and G. M. White. Dordrecht: Reidel.
    1985   "The Once- and Twice-born: Self and Practice among Psychiatrists and Christian Psychiatrists." In *Physicians of Western Medicine: Anthropological Approaches to Theory and Practice,* ed. R. Hahn and A. Gaines. Dordrecht: Reidel.

GEERTZ, CLIFFORD
    1976   "From the Native's Point of View: On the Nature of Anthropological Understanding." In *Meaning in Anthropology,* ed. K. H. Basso and H. A. Selby. Albuquerque: University of New Mexico Press.

GOFFMAN, ERVING
  1961   *Asylums: Essays on the Social Situations of Mental Patients and Other Inmates.* New York: Doubleday.

GOOD, MARY-JO DELVECCHIO
  1985   "Discourses on Physician Competence." In *Physicians of Western Medicine.* Dordrecht: D. Reidel.

GROB, GERALD N.
  1966   *The State and the Mentally Ill: A History of Worcester State Hospital in Massachusetts, 1830–1920.* Durham, N.C.: University of North Carolina Press.
  1973   *Mental Institutions in America: Social Policy to 1875.* New York: Free Press.
  1983   *Mental Illness and American Society 1875–1940.* New York: Princeton University Press.

HAHN, ROBERT A.
  1985   "A World of Internal Medicine: Portrait of an Internist." In *Physicians of Western Medicine: Anthropological Approaches to Theory and Practice,* ed. R. Hahn and A. Gaines. Dordrecht: Reidel.

HALEY, JAY
  1984   *Ordeal Therapy: Unusual Ways to Change Behavior.* San Francisco: Jossey-Bass.

HARAWAY, DONNA
  1988   "Situated Knowledges: The Science Question in Feminism and the Privilege of Partial Perspective." *Feminist Studies* 14(3):575–599.

HARRE, ROM
  1980   *Social Being: A Theory for Social Psychology.* Totowa, N.J.: Littlefield, Adams and Company.

HARVEY, DAVID
  1985   *Consciousness and the Urban Experience.* Baltimore: Johns Hopkins University Press.
  1985   *The Urbanization of Capital.* Baltimore: Johns Hopkins University Press.
  1989   *The Condition of Postmodernity.* Oxford: Blackwell.

HIRSCHMAN, ALBERT O.
  1977   *The Passions and the Interests: Political Arguments for Capitalism Before Its Triumph.* Princeton, N.J.: Princeton University Press.

HOPPER, KIM
  1988   "More Than Passing Strange: Homelessness and Mental Illness in New York City." *American Ethnologist* 15(1):155–167.

HOPPER, KIM, and JILL HAMBURG
  1984   *The Making of America's Homeless: From Skid Row to New Poor, 1945–1984.* New York: Community Service Society.

IGNATIEFF, MICHAEL
  1983   "State, Civil Society and Total Institutions: A Critique of Recent Social Histories of Punishment." In *Social Control and the State: Historical and Comparative Essays,* ed. S. Cohen and A. Scull. Oxford: Martin Robertson.

INGLEBY, DAVID
    1980   "Understanding 'Mental Illness'." In *Critical Psychiatry,* ed. David Ingleby. New York: Pantheon Books.
    1982   "The Social Construction of Mental Illness." In *The Problem of Medical Knowledge: Examining the Social Construction of Medicine.* Edinburgh: Edinburgh University Press.
    1983   "Mental Health and Social Order." In *Social Culture and the State: Historical and Comparative Essays,* ed. S. Cohen and A. Scull. Oxford: Martin.

JONES, KATHLEEN
    1979   "Deinstitutionalization in Context." *Milbank Memorial Fund Quarterly/ Health and Society* 57(4):552–569.
    1982   "Scull's Dilemma." *British Journal of Psychiatry* 141:221–226.

KELLEY, JAMES G.
    1973   "Antidote for Arrogance: Training for Community Psychology." In *Community Mental Health: Social Action and Reaction,* ed. Bruce Denner and Richard H. Price. New York: Holt, Rinehart, and Winston, Inc.

KLEINMAN, ARTHUR
    1988   *Re-thinking Psychiatry: From Cultural Category to Personal Experience.* New York: Free Press.

KLERMAN, GERALD L.
    1977   "Better But Not Well: Social and Ethical Issues in the De-institutionalization of the Mentally Ill." *Schizophrenia Bulletin* 3(4):617–631.

KONNER, MELVIN
    1987   *Becoming a Doctor: A Journey of Initiation in Medical School.* New York: Viking.

KOVEL, J.
    1980   "The American Mental Health Industry." In *Critical Psychiatry,* ed. David Ingleby. New York: Pantheon.

LAKOFF, GEORGE, and MARK JOHNSON
    1980   *Metaphors We Live By.* Chicago: University of Chicago Press.

LANDY, DAVID
    1982   "On Anthropology and the Deinstitutionalization of Psychiatric Patients." *Medical Anthropology Newsletter* 13(4):3–4.

LENTRICCHIA, FRANK
    1988   *Ariel and the Police: Michel Foucault, William James, Wallace Stevens.* Madison: The University of Wisconsin Press.

LEVINE, MURRAY
    1981   *The History and Politics of Community Mental Health.* Oxford: Oxford University Press.

LIGHT, DONALD
    1980   *Becoming Psychiatrists: The Professional Transformation of Self.* New York: W. W. Norton.

MAHLER, MARGARET
    1975   *The Psychological Birth of the Human Infant: Symbiosis and Individuation.* New York: Basic Books.

MAIN, T. F.
1957   "The Ailment." *British Journal of Medical Psychology*, 30, 129–145.

MARRIOTT, MCKIM
1955   "Little Communities in an Indigenous Civilization." In *Village India*, ed. by M. Marriott. Chicago: University of Chicago Press.

MARTIN, LUTHER H., HUCK GUTMAN, and PATRICK H. HUTTON
1988   *Technologies of the Self: A Seminar with Michel Foucault*. Amherst: University of Massachusetts Press.

MATTHEWS, DARYL B.
1980   *Disposable Patients: Situational Factors in Emergency Psychiatric Decisions*. Lexington, Mass.: Lexington Books.

MERTON, DON, and GARY SCHWARTZ
1982   "Metaphor and Self: Symbolic Process in Everyday Life." *American Anthropologist* 84:796–810.

MIZRAHI, TERRY
1986   *Getting Rid of Patients: Contradictions in the Socialization of Physicians*. New Brunswick, N.J.: Rutgers University Press.

MOLLICA, RICHARD F.
1983   "From Asylum to Community: The Threatened Disintegration of Public Psychiatry." *New England Journal of Medicine* 308(7):367–373.

MUMFORD, EMILY
1970   *Interns: From Students to Physicians*. Cambridge, Mass.: Harvard University Press.

ORTNER, SHERRY B.
1984   "Theory in Anthropology Since the Sixties." *Comparative Studies in Society and History* 26(1):126–166.

PRATT, MARY LOUISE
1986   "Fieldwork in Common Places." In *Writing Culture: The Poetics and Politics of Ethnography*, ed. J. Clifford and G. Marcus. Berkeley, Los Angeles, London: University of California Press.

READ, KENNETH E.
1980   *Other Voices*. New York: Chandler and Sharp.

REYNOLDS, DAVID K., and N. L. FARBEROW
1977   *Endangered Hope: Experiences in Psychiatric Aftercare Facilities*. Berkeley: University of California Press.

RHODES, LORNA A.
1984   "'This Will Clear Your Mind': The Use of Metaphors for Medication in Psychiatric Settings." *Culture, Medicine and Psychiatry* 8:49–70.

RITTENBERG, WILLIAM
1985   "Mary; Patient as Emergent Symbol on a Pediatrics Ward: The Objectification of Meaning as Social Process." In *Physicians of Western Medicine: Anthropological Approaches to Theory and Practice*, ed. R. Hahn and A. Gaines. Dordrecht: Reidel.

ROTHMAN, DAVID J.
1971   *The Discovery of the Asylum: Social Order and Disorder in the New Republic*. Boston: Little, Brown and Co.

1980   *Conscience and Convenience: The Asylum and Its Alternatives in Progressive America*. Boston: Little, Brown and Co.

1983   "Social Control: The Uses and Abuses of the Concept in the History of Incarceration." In *Social Control and the State: Historical and Comparative Essays*, ed. S. Cohen and A. Scull. Oxford: Martin Robertson.

SACKS, OLIVER
1984   *A Leg to Stand On*. New York: Harper and Row.

SANFORD, JOHN A.
1977   *Healing and Wholeness*. New York: Paulist Press.

SCHEFF, THOMAS J.
1966   *Being Mentally Ill: A Sociological Theory*. Chicago: Aldine.

SCHEINFELD, DANIEL, and PATRICIA MARSHALL
n.d.   "The Study of Emotions as an Approach to Understanding Culture." Unpublished manuscript.

SCHEPER-HUGHES, NANCY
1981   "Dilemmas in Deinstitutionalization: A View from Inner City Boston." *Journal of Operational Psychiatry* 12(2):90–99.

1982   "Anthropologists and the 'Crazies': Recent Work in Cultural Psychiatry." *Medical Anthropology Newsletter* 13(2):1–2, 6–11.

SCHÖN, DONALD
1983   *The Reflective Practitioner: How Practitioners Think in Action*. New York: Basic Books.

SCHUTZ, DONALD
1967   *Collected Papers I: The Problem of Social Reality*. Ed. M. Natanson. The Hague: Martinus Nijhoff.

SCULL, ANDREW T.
1979   *Museums of Madness: The Social Organization of Insanity in Nineteenth-Century England*. London: Allen Lane.

1981a   "Progressive Dreams, Progressive Nightmares: Social Control in 20th Century America." *Stanford Law Review* 33(3):575–590.

1981b   "The New Trade in Lunacy: The Recommodification of the Mental Patient." *American Behavioral Scientist* 24(6):741–754.

1983   "Humanitarianism or Control? Some Observations on the History of Anglo American Psychiatry." In *Social Control and the State: Historical and Comparative Essays*, ed. S. Cohen and A. Scull. Oxford: Martin Robertson.

1984   *Decarceration: Community Treatment and the Deviant: A Radical View*, 2nd ed. Cambridge: Polity Press.

SEARLES, HAROLD F.
1967   "The 'Dedicated Physician' in Psychotherapy and Psychoanalysis." In *Crosscurrents in Psychiatry and Psychoanalysis*, ed. Robert Gibson. New York: Lippincott.

SEGAL, STEVEN, JIM BAUMOHL, and ELSIE JOHNSON
1977   "Falling through the Cracks: Mental Disorder and Social Margin in a Young Vagrant Population." *Social Problems* 24:387–400.

SHAH, SALEEM A.
1982   "Dangerousness and Civil Commitment of the Mentally Ill: Some Public Policy Considerations." In *Psychiatry and Ethics: Insanity, Ra-*

tional Autonomy and Mental Health Care, ed. Rem B. Edwards. Buffalo, New York: Prometheus Books.

SHARAF, MYRON, and DANIEL LEVINSON
1964   "The Quest for Omnipotence in Professional Training." *Psychiatry* 27:135–149.

SHEEHAN, SUSAN
1983   *Is There No Place On Earth For Me?* New York: Vintage Books.

SHEM, SAMUEL
1978   *The House of God.* New York: Dell.

SHWEDER, RICHARD, and EDMUND S. BOURNE
1984   "Does the Concept of the Person Vary Cross-Culturally?" In *Cultural Conceptions of Mental Health and Therapy,* ed. A. Marsell and G. White. Dordrecht: Reidel.

SIEGLER, MIRIAM, and HUMPHREY OSMOND
1976   *Models of Madness, Models of Medicine.* New York: Harper and Row.

SOREFF, STEPHEN M.
1981   *Management of the Psychiatric Emergency.* New York: John Wiley and Sons.

STAMM, IRA
1987   "Counter-transference in Hospital Treatment: Basic Concepts and Paradigms." *The Menninger Foundation,* Occasional Paper No. 2.

STARR, PAUL
1982   *The Transformation of American Medicine: The Rise of a Sovereign Profession and the Making of a Vast Industry.* New York: Basic Books.

STEIN, HOWARD F.
1985   *The Psychodynamics of Medical Practice: Unconscious Factors in Patient Care.* Berkeley, Los Angeles, London: University of California Press.

SUDNOW, DAVID
1963   "Normal Crimes: Sociological Features of the Penal Code in a Public Defender Office." *Social Problems* 12:255–276.

SZAZ, THOMAS
1961   *The Myth of Mental Illness.* New York: Harper and Row.

TALLY, TED
1981   *Terra Nova.* New York: Nelson Doubleday.

TAUSSIG, MICHAEL
1980   "Reification and the Consciousness of the Patient." *Social Science and Medicine* 14B:3–13.

TAYLOR, CAROL
1970   *In Horizontal Orbit: Hospitals and the Cult of Efficiency.* New York: Holt, Rinehart and Winston.

THOMPSON, E. P.
1967   "Time, Work-Discipline, and Industrial Capitalism." *Past and Present* 38:56–97.

TRAUBE, ELIZABETH G.
1986   *Cosmology and Social Life: Ritual Exchange Among the Mambai of East Timor.* Chicago: University of Chicago Press.

WAITZKIN, HOWARD
  1983   *The Second Sickness: Contradictions of Capitalist Health Care.* New York: Macmillan.

WARNER, R.
  1985   *Recovery from Schizophrenia: Psychiatry and Political Economy.* London: Routledge and Kegan Paul.

WARREN, CAROL A. B.
  1981   "New Forms of Social Control: The Myth of Deinstitutionalization." *American Behavioral Scientist* 24(6):724–742.

WELLIN, EDWARD, DORIA P. SLESINGER, and C. DAVID HOLLISTER
  1987   "Psychiatric Emergency Services: Evolution, Adaptation and Proliferation." *Social Science and Medicine* 24(6):475–482.

WILSON, HOLLY S.
  1986   "Usual Hospital Treatments in the United States' Community Mental Health System: A Dispatching Process." In *Practice to Grounded Theory in Qualitative Research in Nursing,* ed. W. Carole Chenitz and Janice M. Swanson. Menlo Park, CA: Addison-Wesley.

Index

COMPARATIVE STUDIES OF
HEALTH SYSTEMS AND MEDICAL CARE

For a complete list of titles in this series, please contact the
Sales Department
University of California Press
2120 Berkeley Way
Berkeley, CA 94720

Designer:	Linda M. Robertson
Compositor:	Prestige Typography
Text:	10/12 Baskerville
Display:	Bembo Bold
Printer:	Braun-Brumfield, Inc.
Binder:	Braun-Brumfield, Inc.

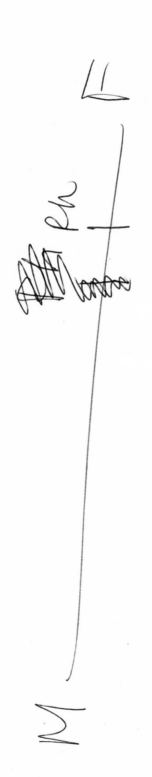